Darko Katić

Situation Interpretation for knowledge- and model based Laparoscopic Surgery

Situation Interpretation for knowledge- and model based Laparoscopic Surgery

by
Darko Katić

KIT Scientific Publishing

Dissertation, Karlsruher Institut für Technologie (KIT)
Fakultät für Informatik

Tag der mündlichen Prüfung: 11. Dezember 2015
Erster Gutachter: Prof. Dr.-Ing. Rüdiger Dillmann
Zweiter Gutachter: Prof. Dr. Rudi Studer
Dritter Gutachter: Dr.-Ing. Stefanie Speidel

Impressum

KIT Scientific Publishing

Karlsruher Institut für Technologie (KIT)
KIT Scientific Publishing
Straße am Forum 2
D-76131 Karlsruhe

KIT Scientific Publishing is a registered trademark of Karlsruhe Institute of Technology. Reprint using the book cover is not allowed.

www.ksp.kit.edu

Print on Demand 2016

ISBN 978-3-7315-0527-3
DOI 10.5445/KSP/1000054609

Situation Interpretation for knowledge- and model based Laparoscopic Surgery

zur Erlangung des akademischen Grades eines

Doktors der Ingenieurswissenschaften

der Fakultät für Informatik
des Karlsruher Instituts für Technologie (KIT)

genehmigte

Dissertation

von

Darko Katić

aus Karlovac

Tag der mündlichen Prüfung: 11.12.2015
Erster Gutachter: Prof. Dr.-Ing. Rüdiger Dillmann
Zweiter Gutachter: Prof. Dr. Rudi Studer
Dritter Gutachter: Dr.-Ing. Stefanie Speidel

Acknowledgements

My time as a research assistant at the Institute for Anthropomatics and Robotics was an amazing and enriching experience. The most memorable aspect are without doubt the people I got the chance to meet and work with. Their great support, criticism and scientific advice was a major component of the success of this thesis.

In particular, I would like to thank Prof. Rüdiger Dillmann for his scientific guidance and for creating a special work environment which allows individuals to thrive and develop their own ideas. Additionally I want to express my gratitude to Prof. Rudi Studer for agreeing to be the second reviewer for my thesis and for the interesting discussions and insights. I would also like to thank Prof. Bernhard Beckert, Prof. Michael Beigl, Prof. Frank Bellosa, Prof. Dennis Hofheinz for joining the examination board.

A very special thank you is dedicated to Dr. Stefanie Speidel. The value of her support, guidance and constructive criticism had great influence on this thesis. Her professional lead of the computer assisted surgery group created opportunities which otherwise would have been unattainable. I thank Yoo-Jin Azad, Sebastian Schalck, Sebastian Bodenstedt and Michael Delles for the unforgettable time in the office and for all the lunches and coffee breaks we spent together. I would also like to especially thank Sebastian Bodenstedt for the sharing of expertise and his invaluable help during night-long experiments full of hardware failures and calibration issues. I also thank Sebastian Röhl and Stefan Suwelack for some great conferences and their consulting of us younger research assistants as well as Enrico Kuhn and Roland Unterhinninghofen for their support and encouragement. A special thanks is reserved for Gunther Sudra who supervised my work as a student and is partially to blame for me getting into academia.

Diane Becker, Isabelle Wappler and Christine Brand of our office team were an incredible help in more than just the administrative processes. I want to thank them for their unshakable patience, knowledge and skill. Especially, I would like to thank Isabelle Wappler for our customary lunches and all the food she shared with me. I also express many thanks to Michael Neaga for his expertise and professional administration of the software infrastructure and the pleasant discussion during the years.

I would also like to express gratitude towards the colleagues of the High Performance Humanoid Technologies department and Prof. Tamim Asfour. A special thanks goes to Ömer Terlemez and Christian Mandery for all the discussions and encouragements. I would also like to thank Sandy Engelhardt and Keno März from the German Cancer Research Center for the great talks, exchange of expertise and shared supervision of student works. Also, I thank Simone Brandstädter from the Psychological Institute of the University of Heidelberg for great talks and insights.

This thesis would have been impossible without the commitment, collaboration and expertise of the minimally invasive surgery group at the University Hospital Heidelberg. My thanks go to Anna-Laura Wekerle for her direct impact on the thesis through her medical expertise. Furthermore I would like to thank Hannes Kenngott for ingenious ideas, suggestions and for having an unmatchable sense for the scientific process. I would also like to thank Martin Wagner for his incredible dedication and commitment.

My time as a research assistant offered me the privilege to mentor many great and gifted students. I thank all of them for their hard work, great questions and invaluable contributions to this thesis. In particular, I thank Sebastian Löfflath, Jochen Görtler, Patrick Spengler, Jürgen Schuck, Nicolas Dürr, Richard Fallert, Fabian Gärtner, Socrates Ponce, Tobias Christian, Thomas Weicker, Julia Reinsch, Vera Genten, Isabel Funke, Oliver Neumann, Arthur Derathe, Rihards Kolkovskis, Chantal Julliard, Roman Ungefuk and Marko Stankovic.

I express my deepest gratitudes to all my friends and my family for their support and patience. In particular, I thank my parents Nada and Darko and my aunt Mirjana for all the have done for me. Above all, I thank my beloved wife Isabelle.

Abstract

Image guided and computer assisted surgeries are increasingly becoming a reality in clinics. Assistance systems, supporting surgeons with additional information such as images, sensor data and visualizations of patient information as well as intervention plans or even robotic support are certain to become integral to surgical workflows in the future. Yet, they have the potential to overload the surgeon and turn him into an administrator of software systems. At their worst, they make his job more difficult.

To avoid this problem of information overflow, new man-machine interfaces are necessary. For this purpose, context-aware systems are very promising. They are to act as automatic information filters which pick out the important and currently relevant bits of information from the available data. This enables targeted assistance during the entire surgery.

Such context-aware systems need to be knowledgeable. They need profound knowledge to appropriately and reliably react to developing events during the surgery. However, being knowledgeable is not enough. As with a human assistant with just formal education, a system without experience will likely have issues in uncommon, special situations. Therefore the application of formal and experience-based knowledge for the task of intraoperative recognition of surgical phases is explored in this work. In doing so, contributions to the following fields were made: representation of formal as well as experience-based knowledge, knowledge-based situation interpretation and context-aware Augmented Reality.

The representation of formal knowledge, as found in books or taught in lectures, is realized using Description Logics formalized in the Ontology Web Language. As part of this thesis, two different ontologies (The Ontology for Laparascopy and LapOntoSPM) were created to capture all knowledge relevant for the interpretation of laparascopic procedures. This representation is used to represent actual surgeries with a high degree of fidelity in a semantic way, thus expressing experience-based knowledge. For this purpose, the vocabulary provided by the ontologies is used. This links and integrates both knowledge types.

The idea behind the situation interpretation is to recognize the current phase of the surgery so that just the currently appropriate information is delivered. Methodically, this work focuses on formal knowledge, experience-based knowledge and combinations thereof.

Formal knowledge by medical experts about phases is captured with rules. Several rule languages are examined for this. To make use of experience, Random Forests are used to recognize the current phase and nGrams to predict future occurrences in the OR. To extend the formal approach, swarm-optimization to learn rules from experience-based knowledge is used. These rules can then be refined, corrected and extended as necessary by medical experts. To incorporate formal knowledge into machine learning, a Composition of Random Forests is used. The idea is to take advantage of formal knowledge about possible transitions between phases to simplify the recognition process and distribute it over multiple Random Forests.

An important part of this contribution is the assessment of the quality of the proposed algorithms in a systematic, repeatable fashion. For this purpose, manual annotations of surgeries are used. To evaluate robustness, the input data is distorted in a reasonable fashion to simulate noisy sensors. This allows realistic assessment of the algorithms. Furthermore, two different surgery types (adrenalectomies and pancreas resections) are used to evaluate the ability to generalize.

To show the applicability to real-world scenarios, two clinically relevant phantom experiments in laparascopy and dental implant surgery were conducted. For this purpose, Augmented Reality visualizations were developed and integrated into MediAssist, a system for image guided surgery. In laparascopy, vital information, e.g. about targets (e.g. tumors) and vital structures (e.g. veins) are visualized. The Augmented Reality for this case is displayed in endoscopic images, the view surgeons are already accustomed to. For dental implants, visual assistance about the correct placing and aligning of the dental bur in the mandible is presented. The visualizations are shown using a head mounted display to fit in the established workflow. All visualizations are activated depending on the context using the phase recognized via situation interpretation.

Kurzfassung

Rechnergestützte Chirurgie drängt immer stärker in den klinischen Alltag. Assistenzsysteme, die Chirurgen durch zusätzliche Information helfen, sind ein wichtiger Bestandteil der Zukunft der Chirurgie. Diese Entwicklung trägt jedoch auch die inhärente Gefahr, Chirurgen mit Information zu überfordern. Der Chirurg droht zu einem Verwalter von Softwaresystemen zu werden. Im schlimmsten Fall wird so seine Arbeit sogar erschwert.

Um dem Problem der Informationsüberflutung Herr zu werden sind neue Mensch-Machine-Schnittstellen notwendig. Kontext-bezogenen Systeme sind hierzu ein vielversprechender Ansatz. Sie dienen als automatische Informationsfilter, welche die aktuell relevanten Informationen aus der Datenflut extrahieren und eine gezielte Unterstützung der OP realisieren.

Kontext-bezogene Systeme müssen über Wissen verfügen, um angemessen und zuverlässig auf die Entwicklungen während der Operation zu reagieren. Das allein ist aber nicht ausreichend. Wie bei einem menschlichen Assistenten, der nur über eine formale Ausbildung verfügt, wird ein System ohne Erfahrungswissen Probleme in ungewöhnlichen Ausnahmesitation haben. In dieser Arbeit wird deshalb das Spannungsfeld zwischen formalem Wissen und Erfahrungswissen untersucht. Dabei werden Beiträge in der Repräsentation von formalem Wissen, der Repräsentation von erfahrungsbasiertem Wissen, der wissensbasierten Situationserkennung und der kontext-bezogenen Erweiterten Realität geleistet.

Die Repräsentation von formalem Wissen, wie es in Büchern und medizinischen Vorlesungen zu finden ist, erfolgt über Beschreibungslogiken in der Ontology Web Language. Dazu wurden zwei Ontologien entwickelt: The Ontology for Laparascopy und LapOntoSPM (Ontology for Surgical Process Models in Laparoscopy). Sie umfassen das gesamte formale Wissen um laparaskopische Situationen zu erfassen und werden verwendet um tatsählich durchgeführte Operationen semantisch darzustellen. Ziel ist die Abbildung von Erfahrungswissen über die Annotierung chirurgischer Abläufe mit dem Vokabular der Ontologie. So werden formales Wissen und Erfahrungswissen verbunden und integriert.

Die Grundidee ist es die aktuelle Phase der Operation zu erkennen. So kann direkt die Informationsfilterung stattfinden. Methodisch wird dabei formales Wissen, Erfahrungswissen sowie deren Kombination verwendet.

Formales Wissen medizinscher Experten über die Phasen wird mit Regeln erfasst. Dazu wurden diverse Regelsprachen betrachtet und verglichen. Erfahrungswissen wirds mittels eines lernbasierten Verfahrens, Random Forests, umgesetzt. nGramme werden für die intraoperative Vorhersage von Ereignissen verwendet. Zur Kombination werden zwei Ansätze verfolgt. Der formale Ansatz wird mittels Schwarmoptimierung erweitert. Die Idee ist, Regeln mit Hilfe von Lernverfahren aus Erfahrungswissen zu extrahieren. Diese können dann von medizinischen Experten verifiziert, korrigiert und erweitert werden. Um formales Wissen in den erfahrungsbasierten Ansatz zu bringen wurde ein neues Verfahrens basierend auf einer sog. Komposition aus Random Forests entwickelt. Dabei wird formales Wissen über mögliche Phasenabfolgen genutzt, um die Erkennung zu vereinfachen und auf mehrere Random Forests zu verteilen.

Ein wichtiger Beitrag ist die systematische, wiederholbare Evaluation der Algorithmen. Dazu wurden manuelle Annotationen echter Operationen verwendet. Um die Robustheit realistisch zu evaluieren, wurden die Evaluationsdaten künstlich verrauscht. Zusätzlich wurde die Evaluation auf zwei Eingriffstypen (Gallenblasenentfernung und Pankreasresektion) durchgeführt um die Verallgemeinerungsfähigkeit zu untersuchen.

Um die Anwendbarkeit des Ansatzes auf reale Probleme und Szenarien zu untersuchen wurden klinisch relevante Experimente in der Laparaskopie und Dentalimplantologie durchgeführt. Zu diesem Zweck wurden Visualisierungen mittels Erweiterter Realität entworfen und die Phasenerkennung an MediAssist, einem System für die bildbasierte Chirurgie, angebunden. Im laparaskopischem Fall wurden Informationen, etwa über Ziel- und Vitalstrukturen (Tumore, Venen,...) direkt auf den Endoskopbildern dargestellt. Für das Setzen von Dentalimplantaten wurden visuelle Hilfen zum Positionieren des Bohrers angezeigt. Dazu wurde ein Durchsichtbrillensystem verwendet. Alle Visualisierungen werden in Abhängigkeit der erkannten Phase ein- und ausgeblendet und sind somit kontext-bezogen.

Contents

List of Figures

List of Tables

1. Introduction

Image guidance and computer assisted interventions are becoming increasingly common. Assistance systems, which aid the surgeon by providing additional information in the form of images, measurements and visualizations of preoperative planing data or even robotic support are bound to become an integral part of surgical workflows in the future. However, they have the potential to overwhelm the surgeon and turn him into an administrator of software systems. At their worst, they make his job more difficult. Even rather simple virtual images displayed on top of the patient's anatomy are shown to distract so much that surgeons are more likely to miss important events [10]. With more advanced assistance systems, it will be rather difficult to find the relevant bits of information in the sea of data.

The quantitative and qualitative availability of information is a very promising step towards better patient care. In the past, surgeons had little to rely on except themselves, their knowledge, experience and assistants. Thus the success of the surgery depended largely on the experience and the skills of the surgeon. Computer assistance during the intervention, on the other hand, is intended to improve patient care by extensive computer-based support of the manual and decision making skills of the surgeon. This corresponds to "Intelligence Amplification" as described by Skagestad [50]. At its core, the idea is that surgeons with computer assistance perform better than surgeons alone. In fact, even simple visualizations or warnings, generated at the right time, can have great effects on patient outcome.

Yet, it is evident, that picking up the right information in a working environment as shown in Fig.1.1 is difficult. This increase of information adds complexity to the operating room. Surgeons can no longer focus solely on the patient and the intervention itself. They also need to manage assisting devices and process additional data. These additional activities

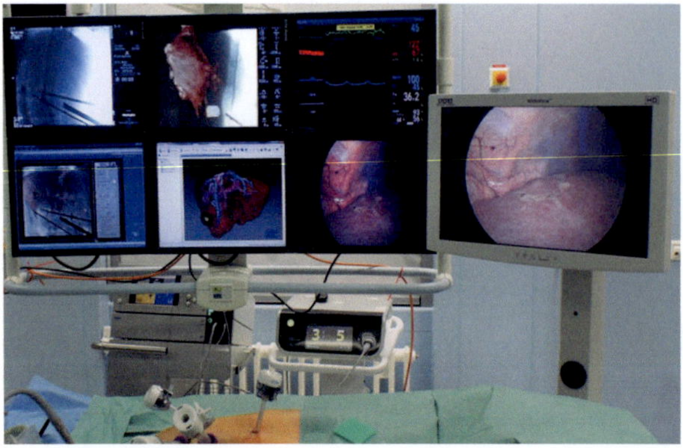

Figure 1.1.: Visualization and information representation which can cause information overflow intraoperatively

should not extend the duration of the surgery. This may cause severely adverse effects. Human capabilities to process and interpret the data [62] can easily be exceeded, increasing the cognitive load to unsustainable levels. At this point data is "physically available" but "not operationally effective" [17]. Important bits of information may be missed and even get actively ignored as a means of coping with the information overload. At worst, the actions of the assistance system can degenerate into unwanted distractions. The assistance systems then simply stop being useful. In the already stressful environment of an OR the effects of cognitive overload are amplified. In particular, image-guided surgery can considerably increase the visual complexity of a scene when not used with care.

To exploit the potential of computer assisted surgery, new strategies of interaction with assistance systems need to be explored. Manual adjustment of assistance systems, as it worked well in the past, does not scale with truly computerized surgery. Manual adaption is difficult, time consuming and often completely unfeasible. Especially during time-critical or risky situations it is not an option. The mental effort required to manage visualizations, information displays and robotic systems requires too much focus and distracts from the actual task, i.e. taking care of the patient.

A better solution to this problem of sensory overload is the application of intelligent filters that automatically select the most appropriate action or visualization for the current situation. The need for such adaptive interfaces in surgery is well known and documented in literature [33]. In their review paper [39] Linte et al., emphasize the need for context-awareness as a means of bringing augmented reality into actual clinical application. They stress "the importance of selecting the most relevant information from the available multimodal imaging data to be displayed to the operator at a particular stage of the procedure". There is even preliminary evidence for detrimental effects of visual assistance functions without context-awareness. It has been shown that, for certain tasks, Augmented Reality can cause "inattentional blindness". Surgeons were shown to be less likely to recognize "unexpected findings" when using Augmented Reality in contrast to an unaugmented view [10]. These examples highlight the importance of context-awareness for medical applications. The development of context-awareness is a crucial step towards bringing advanced assistance systems into clinical practice.

This work therefore focuses on methods for the intraoperative, automatic recognition of the current phase of a surgery. Knowing the phase, it is possible to adapt the assistance accordingly. By defining phases in a way, that each phase is in need of a distinct set of assistance functions, true context-aware assistance is possible.

As stated by Woods et al. [62], the lack of knowledge is a crucial obstacle to understanding. It should thus be part of context-awareness. Like a human assistant, one would expect a context-aware software managing assistance systems on behalf of the surgeon to be "knowledgeable". It needs a profound set of knowledge to appropriately and reliably react to the ongoing events during the surgery. One goal of this work, therefore, is to represent medical knowledge in a generic, reusable way. Examples of sources for this formal knowledge are lectures at universities, books or reports and inputs from medical experts. This representation of formal knowledge is applied to the task of intraoperative situation interpretation.

However, formal knowledge is not enough. As a human assistant with just formal education, a system that makes only use of formal knowledge is only of limited benefit in uncommon, special situations. A lot of human behavior is intuitive action guided by experience.

This work explores formal knowledge and experience-based knowledge in terms of their use in situation interpretation. Specifically, it is intended to research how interpretation algorithms can make use of formal knowledge, experience and a combination of both.

The ability to interpret ongoing situations is at the core of context-awareness. It enables a formal understanding of the current situation during the surgery. The goal is to give the system the capability of situational awareness, in the sense of "knowing what is going on so you can figure out what to do" as defined by Adam et al in [1]. The "figuring out what to do" part addresses the question of how to manage assistance functions, the "knowing what is going on" is concerned with interpreting the current situation and raising it to a higher level of granularity, namely that of so called phases.

More precisely, a perception component is assumed as given. Thus intraoperative information about the current scene and representation primitives in the form of activities, as discussed in 3.3 is assumed to be available. In practice, such techniques are still parts of ongoing research, for instance by Speidel et al. [52]. These inputs are used to create a model of the situation. This model is analyzed by a situation interpretation algorithm to infer the current surgery phase. This way, a higher-level, more abstract view of the scene is obtained. The term "phase" is currently not used consistently throughout the community. Therefore, this work takes on a pragmatic approach: phases are defined as sections of the surgical procedure in need of a distinct set of assistance functions. Thus context-aware assistance can be provided once the phase is recognized.

As one would expect from a human assistant, the system is to use experience and formal knowledge for this purpose. In this work, rules are used to capture formal knowledge. The rules are used to check whether the model of the situation satisfies given conditions which are indicating a phase. This way the formal knowledge can be applied to recognize phases. Several rule languages have been investigated for this purpose.

However, since some of the knowledge about phases is tacit, i.e. difficult to formalize, experience-based knowledge is also necessary. It is represented by manually annotated surgical workflows. These surgeries are used as input for machine learning, namely the Random Forest algorithm. Another medically relevant application of the situation interpretation is to predict which activities are likely to occur next. This is a very fine-grained problem with many different possibilities. The problem involves more uncertainty than phase recognition. For medical experts, it is very difficult to articulate and enumerate all possible follow-up activities. Therefore, experience-based knowledge is used. This is realized using nGrams, a method for statistical prediction of events based on previously observed ones. To combine these complementary approaches two methods are examined.

To augment the formal knowledge based approach with experience, rules are extracted from annotated surgeries. The idea is to formalize the parts relevant for situation interpretation into an explicit, human-readable form. This captures tacit knowledge, given that it is implicitly contained in the experience. The resulting rules can be verified, extended and corrected by medical experts if necessary. Experience-based knowledge is transferred to formal knowledge, as it is made explicit and formalized. Methodically, swarm optimization is used for this purpose.

To augment experience with formal knowledge, the idea of Compositions of Random Forests has been developed in this work. They exploit formal knowledge about possible transitions of phases given by the surgery plan. The strategy is to partition the task of phase recognition over multiple Random Forests. This way each Random Forest only has to deal with a limited number of phases.

Since all of these situation interpretation approaches rely on knowledge in some way or other, they are called knowledge based interpretation algorithms. This knowledge-based approach raises a number of scientific questions about the representation of knowledge, interpretation of surgical processes and means of providing context-aware assistance. These are detailed in the following.

1.1. Research Questions

As illustrated in chapter 2, most approaches in current literature to context-awareness rely on a mix of feature extraction techniques and machine learning methods to recognize the context. There is no significant emphasis on sophisticated knowledge representation.

Consequently, the proposed algorithms rely on machine learning and training data to learn what medical experts already know. This is a problem because training data is difficult to obtain while formal knowledge from medical literature and surgical experts is already available in different modalities. It is therefore worthwhile to explore how this knowledge can be represented and utilized.

This work therefore focuses on methods for knowledge representation and algorithms which make use of knowledge to recognize the context of the surgery. The research is guided by the following research questions.

- **How can formal surgical knowledge be represented in a reusable and generic way?** Medicine is a huge field with an incredible amount of accumulated knowledge. It has a long tradition of efforts to standardize medical knowledge, naming conventions and procedures. There is also a large amount of medical knowledge representations available, such as SNOMED-CT[1].

  Therefore it is reasonable to attempt to also formalize surgeries in a generic way. The value of such a formalization is not only in the application to context-awareness. The aspect of reusability is also of special importance. It allows other projects and research groups to benefit from the modeled knowledge as it can be used in different settings for different purposes.

  What makes this question difficult is the issue of representing a diverse set of knowledge in a common representational formalism. It is not sufficient to just capture the essence of the knowledge. It also needs to happen in a generic, non-proprietary way to ensure that the knowledge is sharable.

- **How can experienced-based knowledge be represented and linked with formal knowledge so both knowledge types are used in conjunction?** Formal knowledge is insufficient to solve all problems of context-awareness. Experience of actual, observed surgeries needs to be incorporated as well. However, as in human cognition, formal knowledge and experience are not independent. It is obvious that people who have of firm grasp of formal knowledge and a great amount of experience tend to perform very well. Thus the representations of both knowledge types should be compatible

[1] http://www.ihtsdo.org/snomed-ct/

and so they can benefit from each other. The inherent challenge is to combine both knowledge types in a common representation.

- **How can situation interpretation be implemented with the help of formal knowledge, experience-based knowledge and combinations thereof?** Being knowledgeable and experienced is without doubt a useful trait in human assistants. However, it needs to be researched whether this idea also applies to the automatic interpretation of situations to infer the current phase. Most current approaches to context-awareness rely on machine learning, and thus on experience-based knowledge. This work focuses on the question whether the problem of situation interpretation is made easier by including formal knowledge.

  To answer this question is to develop novel interpretation algorithms which make use of formal and experience-based knowledge, as well as a combination thereof to facilitate the recognition of surgical phases.

- **How can situation interpretation methods be applied to provide context-aware assistance in laparascopy and dental implant surgery?** The research is of little value, if it cannot be transferred into the OR. The applicability of the system is shown by two different assistance systems for image guidance in laparascopy and dental implant surgery. The image guidance is realized via Augmented Reality methods.

  What makes this problem difficult is the need for integration of the recognition into the infrastructure of a computer assisted surgery system and the real-time constraints imposed by the application.

1.2. Goals and Contribution

The contributions of this thesis are directly derived from the research question. To find a reasonable and generic solution, it is necessary to develop a knowledge-based system which provides context-aware assistance. In doing so, contributions to the following fields are made: knowledge representation, interpretation and context-aware assistance, as shown in

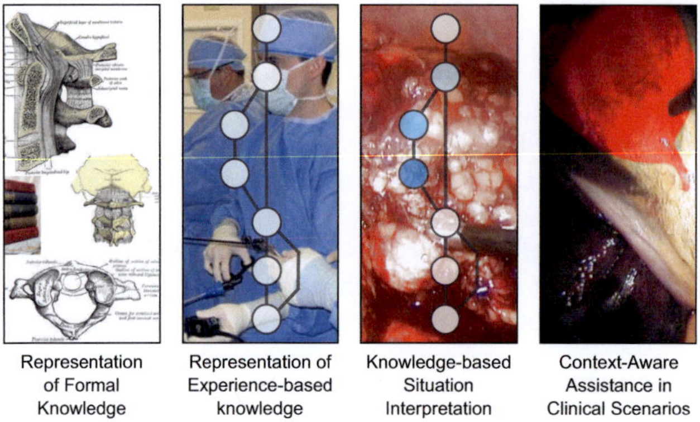

Figure 1.2.: Main areas of contribution of this thesis

Fig.1.2. Additionally the work has to be evaluated in regards of the eventual medical merit. These aspects are further elaborated in the following.

- **Representation of formal knowledge** The representation of formal knowledge is concerned with the formalization of generic medical knowledge as documented in books or presented in lectures. This is limited to the sub-set of knowledge relevant to intraoperative situation interpretation. Specifically, it includes information about the applied instruments (e.g. scalpel, coagulator,...), their functions (e.g. to cut, to coagulate) and the relations between them (e.g. being of a common category *tissue resection instrument*). It is also concerned with knowledge about anatomical structure (e.g. gallbladder, liver,...) which are affected during the surgery and ultimately the actions surgeons can perform with the instruments on the structures (e.g. cutting, dissecting...). The triplet of instrument, action and affected structure is referred to as an activity.

  Apart from these tangible features, knowledge about the surgical process itself needs to be modeled. This concerns for instance the possible transitions of surgical phases (e.g. resection of an organ) or the composition of phases from lower-grained activities (e.g. holding the organ with a grasper, clipping some blood vessel with the clipper and other activities necessary to resect the organ). This is the computational representation of formal knowledge.

The representation cannot happen in arbitrary ways. Apart from content, there are strong formal requirements. The representation is to be reusable and useful in different settings. Thus, no restricted, problem-specific solution is sufficient, but one that can be used beyond the situation interpretation task. To construct the ontology, methods from knowledge engineering are used. The underlying formalism is based on description logic.

- **Representation of experience-based knowledge** Formal knowledge deals with ideas, and sometimes even idealizations. To represent actual experience, those concepts need to be instantiated.

  The representation of formal knowledge is used to describe actual surgeries with a high degree of fidelity and semantics. The idea is to represent the surgery as a series of phases and activities, along with the utilized instruments and affected anatomical structures. This should yield to a more comprehensible representation of the surgery than, for instance, just a sequence of recorded sensor signals.

  This representation is to use the same vocabulary as defined in the knowledge representation. This is a means of linking both. For instance, if a specific scalpel is used in a surgery, all its functional properties such as its ability to cut can be automatically inferred from the general knowledge about the concept *scalpel*.

  The representation of the surgical process is then used to formalize experience-based knowledge. The experience-based knowledge, as defined in this work, is gained from the observation of performed surgeries. Obviously, the actual performance thereof is also part of the experience of a surgeon. But since the assistance system cannot perform the surgery itself, this kind of experience does not apply.

  Similar to the knowledge representation, formal criteria are imposed. The representation should follow established standards as much as possible and be easy to interchange and share.

- **Knowledge-based Situation Interpretation** The idea is to interpret the representation of the surgical process to gain further insight. Specifically, a model of activities which occurred during the surgery is created. Then higher level phases, which overarch individual activities, are inferred. These activities belong together in a medical sense and lead to a specific sub-goal during the surgery. The phases are defined in such a way that each phase requires a specific assistance. Thus, knowing the phase, it is possible to automatically use the appropriate subset of available information. In this way, the automatic information filtering is realized. The information about which activities occurred is assumed to be known. The detection of activities is outside of the scope of this work.

Methodically, formal knowledge is used to facilitate the recognition of phases. However, as just formal knowledge might not be enough in all circumstances, learning based approaches are investigated. They make use of the experience based knowledge of surgeons. Formal knowledge of medical experts about which activities are specific to a certain phase is to be represented with rules. Several rule languages are to be examined for this purpose. To make use of experience, Random Forest are used to recognize the current phase and nGrams to predict future activities. As a combination of both approaches swarm-optimization is examined to learn rules from experience-based knowledge. These rules can then be refined, corrected and extended as necessary by medical experts with formal knowledge. A Composition of Random Forests is used to incorporate formal knowledge into machine learning.

An important contribution in this regard is the assessment of the quality of the proposed algorithms in a systematic, repeatable fashion. In order to do so, manual annotations of surgeries are used as ground truth data. To deal with the issue of robustness, artificially distorted input data is used. This allows a realistic assessment of the algorithm in the absence of perfect input data. For this purpose quality measures need to be defined according to various requirements and the algorithms need to be compared according to these. Since this work focuses mostly on gallbladder removals and pancreas resections, there is a fair amount of variety. This shows the ability to generalize over multiple surgery types.

- **Context-Aware Augmented Reality Assistance in Laparascopy and Dental Implant Surgery** In light of knowledge of the current phase being known, the appropriate subset of available information can be presented to the surgeon. For this purpose, Augmented Reality visualizations are used. For the laparascopic use-case, mainly targets (e.g. tumors) and vital structures (e.g. veins) are visualized. The Augmented Reality for this use-case is to be displayed in the endoscopic images. This is the view surgeons are already accustomed to and which can be delivered without additional hardware. For dental implants, visual assistance about the correct placing and aligning of the dental bur in the mandible is provided. The visualizations are to be shown using a head mounted display. This is to better fit in the established workflow of the procedure. They are displayed only when necessary using the phase recognized via situation interpretation.

  Lastly, the applicability of the research to actual clinical scenarios is assessed. For this purpose the context-aware assistance visualization is put to use in phantom experiments. In the laparascopic scenario, a resection of the gallbladder is performed on a porcine liver. For dental implants, the drilling of implant positions in the mandible of a porcine skull is performed.

The individual parts of this work and their relationships are illustrated in Fig. 1.3. In broad strokes, methods from knowledge engineering are used to create a representation of formal and experience-based knowledge.

Parts of the formal knowledge are formulated in the form of rules to recognize phases, while the experience-based knowledge is used as input for machine learning based approaches (Random Forests and nGrams). For the combination, Random Forest are augmented with formal knowledge to create a Composition of Random Forests. Swarm-based optimization is used to derive formal knowledge in the form of rules from experience as a second mean of combination.

The classifiers are used to recognize the current phase of the surgery. Depending on the current phase, appropriate Augmented Reality visualizations are chosen, thus creating context-aware assistance.

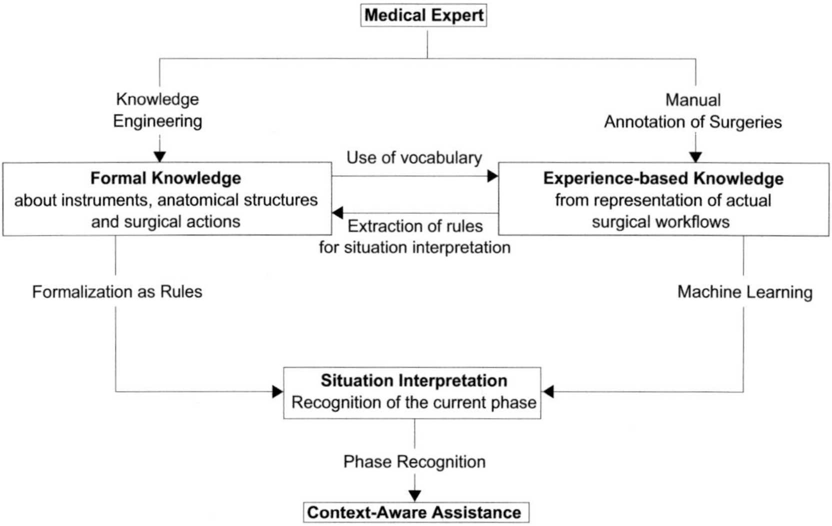

Figure 1.3.: Contributions of this work and their relationship

1.3. Outline

This work is divided in 9 chapters, in line with the goals and contributions. The layout of the chapters is introduced in the following.

- **Chapter 2** This chapter examines the relevant literature in regards to surgical situation interpretation. The reviewed literature is categorized in regards to the level of knowledge formalization.
- **Chapter 3** Here, the means to represent medical knowledge are introduced. The chapter illustrates how to make the system knowledgeable. More specifically, it examines which parts of the domain need to be modeled and which can be omitted since an all encompassing description is impossible. Additionally, formal requirements of the representation formalism are defined. To satisfy partly contradicting requirements, two different ontologies are proposed: The Ontology for Laparascopy and LapOntoSPM. The design decisions and content of both are described in this chapter.

- **Chapter 4** This chapter introduces the algorithms which make use of formal knowledge to recognize the current phase of the surgery. Rule-based interpretation techniques are examined for this purpose. Several rule languages and their aptness for the task, according to specific requirements, are proposed.
- **Chapter 5** The formal approach is contrasted with a experience-based one. Random Forests are used to recognize phases and nGrams to predict up-coming activities.
- **Chapter 6** In this chapter, formal and experience-based knowledge are combined to recognize phases. The Random Forest approach is augmented with formal knowledge to create a Composition of Random Forests. Furthermore, the formal knowledge is extended by generating explicit rules from experience using a swarm-optimization method to find the rules.
- **Chapter 7** In this chapter an image guided removal of the gallbladder with context-aware assistance on a phantom porcine liver is presented. Augmented Reality visualizations of vital structures (the gallbladder and its duct) are displayed only when there is actual danger of harm. Thus safety is improved as warnings are only issued when they are actually relevant and warning fatigue is mitigated.
- **Chapter 8** In addition to the removal of the gallbladder in Chapter 7, an image guided drilling of implant positions in the mandible of a porcine phantom is presented. The currently worked on implant position is automatically recognized and Augmented Reality visualizations are shown to support the work on this drill site.
- **Chapter 9** Here, the thesis as a whole is summarized and discussed. Additionally, an outlook on possible future works is presented.

2. Approaches to Situation Interpretation in Surgery

Several approaches to situation interpretation in surgery have been developed. A noticeable pattern in the current scientific work is the differing degree of knowledge formalization used in the proposed methods. A concise summary of the possible representations can be found in the review article by Lalys et al. [36]. Therefore this is used as a criteria to classify and categorize the numerous approaches to situation interpretation.

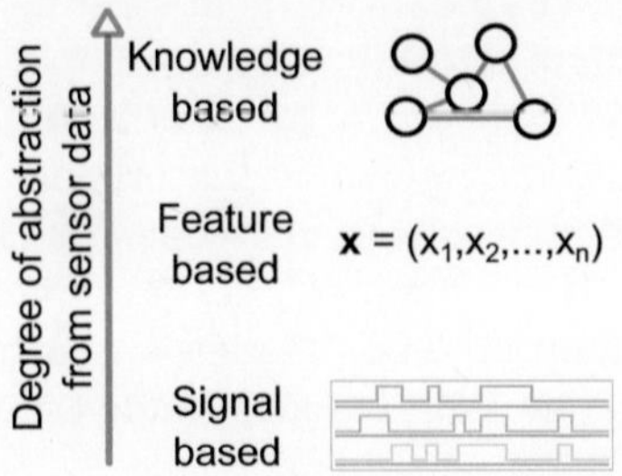

Figure 2.1.: Spectrum of representation strategies based on their level of abstraction.

The categorization is illustrated in Fig. 2.1. On the signal-based end of the spectrum there are approaches which try to operate with as little knowledge and abstraction as possible. They represent surgeries close to the original signals. Interpretation is done via signal processing and machine learning, without further modeling and feature extraction.

Feature-extraction based approaches rely on a higher degree of modeling. In contrast of directly processing the raw data, they extract features and thereby generate models of the situation and the workflow. Sophisticated and established machine learning algorithms are used with these feature vectors to infer the context of the surgery. Usually no new algorithms are developed. Rather established ones are being re-purposed and adapted for the interpretation of workflows.

At the other end of the spectrum are knowledge-based approaches. They rely on a rich, expressive model of the surgery. Integration of medical background knowledge plays a major role in this endeavor. The idea is to create expressive, semantic models of the surgical workflows which are designed to make the interpretation easier.

Examples of these categories are shown in the following and discussed in regards to the work of this thesis.

2.1. Signal-based Approaches

The idea behind this group of algorithms is to directly recognize the phase of the surgery based on sensor data, without creating explicit models. Blum et al. uses this paradigm to analyze laparoscopic cholecystectomies [5]. They employ horizontal and vertical gradient magnitudes, histograms and the pixel values of scaled versions of the original image as features to describe the data coming from the endoscope. The features are computed for all three RGB and HSV channels, and interpreted to infer the current phase. For the interpretation, two different approaches are evaluated and compared: Dynamic Time Warping and Hidden Markov Models.

An even more radical approach is followed by Suzukit et al. [57]. Their idea is to incorporate as little knowledge as possible and infer information about the surgical phase using non-semantic signal processing. They aim to record "all audio visual information in the operating room without any dead angle". As input data, they use a bird-eye view of the operating room from different angles as shown in Fig.2.2 in addition to intraoperative audio signals. Their use-case is in neurosurgery. The audio information includes speech as well as alarm tones and other occurrences in the OR.

To interpret this data, it is assumed that the amount of movement in the OR is indicative of a phase change. To quantify the amount of movement, they do not rely on tracking and recognition methods, but on video file size. The idea is that compression algorithms, which take the temporal neighbors of individual frames into account will be more effective when subsequent video frames are similar. On the contrary, the encoding will be bigger in size for sequences where individual frames differ a lot since in this case there is less redundancy to exploit. Their reasoning therefore is that sections with greater file size indicate movement and change in the OR. A similar idea is applied to analyze the audio signal. The assumption is that a significant increase or decrease in amplitude is indicative of a phase change, since normal chatter is interrupted at these points. For detection Suzuki et al. have identified a frequency band where the chatter takes place and analyze it to find said changes.

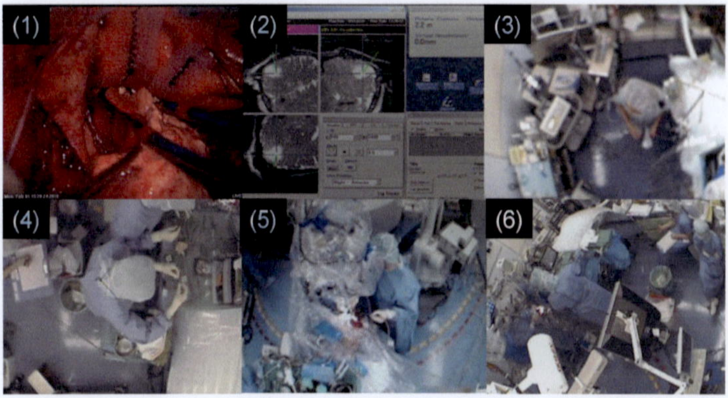

Figure 2.2.: Input data for workflow analysis by Suzuki et al. (1) microscope footage (2) surgical navigation system (3) anesthetist (4) scrub nurse (5) bird-eye view from ceiling above patient, (6) bird-eye view from ceiling above navigation system [57]

2.2. Feature-based Approaches

The idea behind feature-based approaches is to find a suitable set of features and subsequently use established machine learning approaches to relate the feature vector to the surgical phase. Currently, mostly Hidden Markov Models, Dynamic Time Warping and Support Vector Machines are being used for this purpose.

Lalys et al. compute a semantic signature of microscopic video images to find the phase of cataract surgery [37]. This signature is made of cues obtained by image processing approaches. These do not generalize and need to be adapted for each surgery. In this case, they exploit information about shape, color textures as well as global features. The signature is finally classified using Dynamic Time Warping and Hidden Markov Models. This general system setup is shown in Fig.2.3.

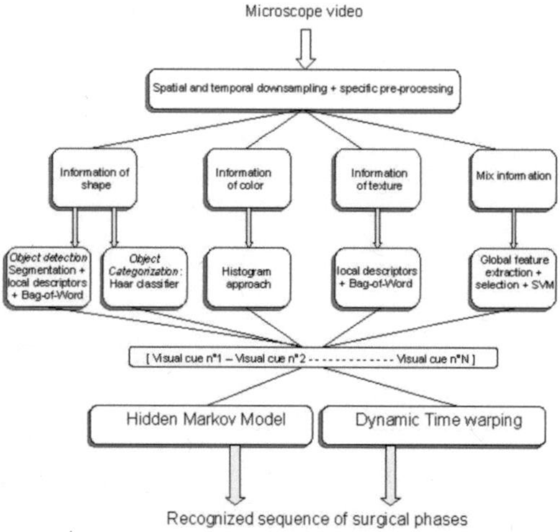

Figure 2.3.: Framework layout used by Lalys et al. [37]

In a similar work Lalys et al. [38] use Support Vector Machines to extract features from microscopic videos of pituitary surgery. Those features are custom-tailored to the surgical type at hand, e.g. they detect the presence of nose retractors or compresses and similar occurrences. After this feature extraction Hidden Markov Models are used to recognize phases.

Bouarfa et al, use a similar approach to interpret laparoscopic cholecystectomies, albeit with a different terminology [6]. For them, a surgery consists of High Level (HLT) and Low Level Tasks (LLT), which roughly corresponds to activities and phases. They aim to recognize HLTs from LLTs. The interpretation is done by Hidden Markov Models. LLTs are binary signals signifying, for instance, whether certain instruments are used or not. This is extracted from video footage. To deal with missing data and noise in the LLTs sequences, Baysians network are used.

Ahmadi et al. aim to create an average surgical workflow from recorded data [2]. Novel surgeries are then mapped to this average procedure using the Dynamic Time Warping algorithm. Phases are inferred by comparison with the average surgery, once they match in the time-domain. The features consist of instrument utilization information.

As a notable alternative to Hidden Markov Models and Dynamic Time Warping, Forestier et al. developed a method based on decision trees to recognize phases of lumbar disk herniation surgeries [11]. They evaluated their approach not only on noise free ground truth data, but also added noise to their evaluation set to judge the robustness of their approach.

Stauder et al. have applied Random Forests for phase recognition in laparoscopic cholecystectomies [53]. As features, they have chosen the used instrument weight irrigation and suction bags, intra-abdominal pressure, inclination of surgical table instruments, HF modes (coagulating and cutting) room light and surgery lamp information. The results were rather mixed as some phases were recognized better than others.

2.3. Knowledge-based Approaches

In contrast to machine learning and even more so, signal processing, the idea behind knowledge-based approaches is to first create a very rich, detailed model of the situation in order to make the interpretation easier.

Franke et al. use surgical situation models to combine a fine-granular detailed representation with context information [12]. Specifically, low-level tasks, high-level tasks, patient status, and the use of medical resource were considered. In contrast to machine learning approaches, where there is usually little more than instrument information, this is a far richer representation of the situation. This model was used in the field of brain tumor removals. With statistical analysis, they estimate the state distribution. They were also able to retrospectively calculate the Viterbi path to correct the estimation postoperatively. This, of course is of no help in online use, but can serve for post-operative purposes

Neumuth et al., also have made tremendous contributions to surgical process modeling. In [42] they take individual process models (iSPM), i.e. semantic annotations of actual surgeries as input. The aim is to compute a statistical mean model, called the generic surgical process model (gSPM). The gSPM can be seen as a formalization of the surgery type in the sense of an accumulation and abstraction of the iSPMs.

Jannin et al. have developed a surgical ontology for neurosurgery with application to the analysis of surgical processes [16], e.g. the generation of postoperative reports and clustering to find similarities between surgeries. As the representational mechanism, they have chosen UML (Unified Modeling Language). It includes a hierarchical model of the workflow. The entire procedure is broken down into a sequence of steps, which consist of individual actions. Actions are described by attributes and affected anatomical structures. This is a clear formalization of the procedure in a well-established language. Yet it is not interconnected with other types of knowledge representations and is more of a proprietary solution.

Lalys et al. also use an ontology to analyze ophthalmological procedures [35]. However, they do not recognize the current phase but rather to use information about the current phase to improve the recognition of activities. The idea is that certain activities only occur during specific phases. The information which activities occur in which phases is modeled in an ontology. It can be used to decrease the complexity of the activity recognition task as the number of activities to be discriminated is limited.

2.4. Discussion

As is evident from the literature review, there is currently a strong bias towards machine learning based methods with sophisticated feature extraction. Most of the work in this area is driven by established algorithms. The contribution is rather in the application and less in the development of novel algorithms. The basic pattern is often similar for machine learning based approaches. Beginning with the raw data, a number of classifiers are used to find descriptive features of the scene which are then used as input for machine learning algorithms.

Signal-based approaches are rather uncommon. When used, the phases are usually defined in a way that suits the underlying data. It has not been shown that the approach generalizes well. The solutions seem to be custom-tailored to the specific task. This as a sign that at least some degree of abstraction and knowledge is necessary, as working on just the raw data is evidently not enough.

It is not trivial to objectively compare the results from each publication. Different surgery types are reported and even for the same type, there is no canonical partition into phases. There are also no publicly available benchmarks. Each research groups works based on their own definitions and data sets. The introduction of formalized models of the surgery helps in this regard. Standards for the representation of surgeries facilitate sharing of data and working on common data sets. This also enables reproducibility of results, a major criteria of scientific work. This issue has been largely recognized in other research domains. However, this is predominately the case in domains like speech or optical character recognition where the representation of data is not problematic [3]. The choice of the representation is often rather straight-forward, where as for surgeries it is not obvious. Coincidentally, machine learning also constrains sharing of knowledge. Knowledge only implicitly embedded in the learned parameters is very difficult to apply to a different use case.

There is no significant work reporting on the use of formal knowledge for situation interpretation. Learning based approaches are dominant. Yet, especially in the medical domain, there are large amounts of formal knowledge available, in the form of books, texts and medical experts. There are many things which can be directly modeled and integrated into the system. It is not necessary to collect and label medical data to have a machine learning based algorithm learn something medical experts already know and can articulate. This is even more of an issue since the labeling of medical data is very time consuming and can, in most cases, only be done by experts. By following the proposed knowledge-based approach, the need for labeled training samples is reduced by incorporating available knowledge directly.

The lack of explicit use of formal knowledge in machine learning also raises safety concerns. The classifiers learned by machine-learning like Support Vector Machines are usually difficult to understand by humans.

The systems act like a black-box. For the surgeon it is not clear under which assumptions the systems operates, what it has learned and what bias the designer of the algorithm introduced when making it (on purpose or unwillingly). Deviation in implicit conceptualizations and definitions can lead to misunderstandings and fundamentally different assessments of the current situation and context. Explicit knowledge representation, like rules, can be understood, verified and corrected by medical experts. Thus, knowledge-based systems act more predictably and surgeons are more likely to accept them in their work space.

Another issue is the flexibility in the way phases are defined. Phases can be defined by simple discrimination criteria. For instance, one could imagine a phase that is characterized by the endoscope being outside of the patient. In this case, even working on the raw endoscopic images can provide decent results. The distinction can be made based on the dominant colors in the image (red of the organs for the inside, green of the sheets for the outside). However, as the complexity of the phases grows, such simple delimiters are more difficult to find. The phase could depend on activities that lie in the past of the surgery or on a combination of factors. For instance, one might want to only issue a warning if a sharp instrument is near a blood vessel. With an appropriate knowledge representation and rule language, a rule can be directly formulated and used to recognize this phase, as shown in chapter 4. Without the knowledge about which anatomical structures are considered "vessels" and which instruments can harm tissues, a learning-based algorithm would need a considerable amount of data to learn which combinations of instruments and anatomical structures warrant a warning and which ones do not. This is not only an example of how the recognition can be facilitated by using formal knowledge. It also shows that it scales better with the complexity of the phases.

A counter-argument to explicit knowledge modeling is that not all knowledge is available directly. Some of it is tacit. Also not all surgeries go according to plan. As already mentioned in chapter 1, machine learning and experience-based knowledge is used to capture variety and deviation from the standard. Furthermore experience-based knowledge is distilled to rules so that special occurrences surgeons might not have considered are automatically found. Also, the robustness of each approach under noisy data is evaluated.

3. Representation of Knowledge for Context Awareness

The purpose of the formal knowledge representation is to capture all formal knowledge necessary to interpret situations in a medically sound way. Specifically, this includes information about instruments, actions and anatomical structures, but also numerical measurements such as distances and mass. It is the kind of formal knowledge that would be found in text books or be taught to medical students. This representation is also used as the vocabulary to represent experience-based knowledge. More specifically, it is used to formulate surgical workflows of actual surgeries to represent experience based knowledge.

To represent the knowledge a representational formalism is necessary. There are numerous formalism available, as evident in the overview by Corcho et al. in [9]. Throughout this thesis OWL (Web Ontology Language), a formalism based on Description Logic (DL) is used. These tools are more thoroughly described in 3.1. The main reason for this choice is that OWL is highly expressive, while still computationally tractable. There is sound support of tools (editors and reasoners). Also, large amounts of medical ontologies in OWL are available for integration and knowledge sharing.

By the goals set in chapter 1 several requirements for the formal knowledge representation are derived. Content-wise there are two requirements:

- **Adequate Completeness** To achieve adequate completeness, the representation needs to be complete in the sense that it entails all information that is required to perform the interpretation task. True completeness cannot be expected, as the domain is far too large. Specifically, the ontology needs to contain information about the instruments, anatomical structures and surgical actions.

Apart from just the enumeration of these entities, relationships are important. For instance, functions of instruments (to cut, to hold...) as well as anatomical properties of organs (being a blood vessel, being attached to some other organ...) should be part of the ontology.

- **Comprehensibility** The representation needs to be comprehensible, i.e. accessible to man and machine alike. The used terminology must be familiar to surgeons and reuse established, well-known ontologies where possible.

Apart from the requirements on the content, there are also technical requirements arising from the needs of practical application.

- **Reusability** The requirement on reusability and facilitated knowledge sharing ensures that the representation of formal knowledge is not an isolated, purpose-specific solution. That is why it is important to reuse other ontologies. This way, the ontology can be integrated with others and aid in other scenarios.
- **Real-time Capability** As the system is to be used for intraoperative context-aware assistance, it needs to run fast enough to deliver an estimate of the current phase in a reasonable time.

It is already evident, that some of the requirements clash. Importing many, large ontologies can have serious impact on the run time performance. The real-time constraints are then easily violated. A reduced, problem specific solution is likely to work faster in practice.

To avoid having to make bad compromises, two different ontologies were developed: "The Ontology for Laparascopy", geared towards performance and "LapOntoSPM" (Laparascopic Ontology for Surgical Process Models) with a strong emphasis on quality and reusability. Both ontologies are connected. The *same as* relation is asserted between the leafs of the inheritance hierarchy. It is thus ensured that, for instance, liver concepts in both ontologies are considered the same. This allows interchangeability of the ontologies.

In the following the terminology used in this thesis is introduced. Then, the key ideas of ontological knowledge representation are outlined. Afterwards, both ontologies are presented.

3.1. Knowledge Representation with Ontologies

The term ontology is used to describe the philosophical attempt to categorize reality. The idea is to formally capture entities (things, ideas, processes...) and their relationships. They are to be categorized hierarchically into groups. To make this possible, a language is necessary to encode such an ontology. Description Logics (DLs) have been developed to serve this purpose. A very detailed introduction to DLs can be found in [4]. In short, DL provides a logical language intended to formalize an ontology. In this thesis, the Web Ontology Language[1] (OWL), a language based on Description Logic is used to author ontologies.

To actually perform reasoning on the knowledge representation and infer facts that are implicitly entailed in the ontology, a so called reasoner is necessary. A reasoner is a software application which infers logical consequences from a set of assertions or axioms, i.e. from an ontology. Examples of reasoners used in this work are FaCT++ [58], HermiT [48] and Pellet [49]. The relation between an ontology, DLs, OWL and reasoners is shown in Fig.3.1.

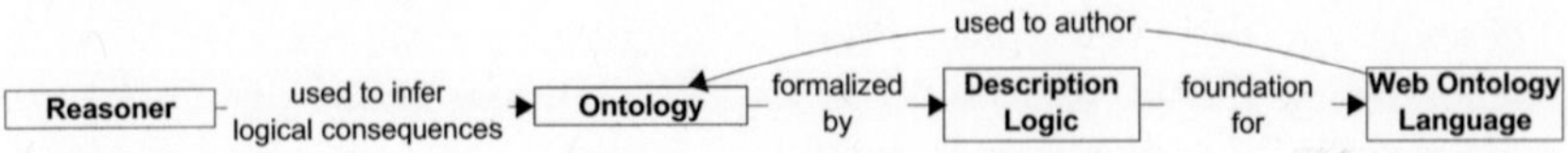

Figure 3.1.: Relationship between ontologies, Description Logic and the Web Ontology Language

An important idea of DLs is the distinction between the TBox (Terminological Box) and Abox (Asserational Box). A TBox describes conceptual knowledge about entities in the world. It is time-invariant, general and not about specific entities. It consists of concepts and relations to describe groups of things. For instance, the general idea of a liver is described by the ontological concept *liver*. Concepts are organized in an inheritance hierarchy. For instance *liver* is defined as a subclass of *organ*. Inheritance is often referred to via the *is-a* relation, denoting the *liver* is a specialization of *organ*. In this work, the *is-a* relation is denoted with $\sqsubseteq$, i.e. *liver* $\sqsubseteq$ *organ*. In the proposed distinction of formal and experience-based knowledge, the TBox corresponds to the formal knowledge.

[1] http://www.w3.org/TR/owl2-overview/

To describe concrete, individual entities, like the liver of a specific patient, the concepts from the TBox need to be instantiated. They are created in the ABox. Here, facts about actual entities are asserted using the concepts and relations. To assert that there is a specific liver of some patient, one would create an instance (or a so called individual) in the ABox by asserting that this instance is an instantiation of the concept *liver*. This is denoted by the assertion *Liver(liver of patient)*, in the syntax *C(i)* whereby *C* represents the name of the concept and *i* the name of the instance. Similarly, an instance of *patient* would be created and both would be connected with the *is body part of* relation. Relation assertion are written as *r(a,b)*, whereby *r* denotes the relation and *a* and *b* the individuals, i.e. *is body part of(liver of patient, patient)*.

Using relations and further concepts additional information can be added to the liver. For instance, it can be asserted that the liver is affected by some surgical instrument at some period in time or that it is diseased in some way. This is done by adding the appropriate assertions to the ABox. The ABox represents concrete activities that have actually occurred. It is thus used to formalize experience-based knowledge.

These are the basic principals of how ontologies are authored with DLs. In the following, the use of these ideas to encode formal knowledge for laprascopy is described. Furthermore the terminology and naming conventions necessary for this are presented.

3.2. Terminology for Surgical Processes

Throughout this manuscript, various terms are used. The following section defines those terms and, where applicable, describe their origin and use in the community.

Surgeries can be viewed at different levels of granularity, ranging from very coarse to highly fine grained. Lalys et al. have defined a standard for granularity levels which is widely accepted [35]. The four main levels are: surgical procedure, phase, step, activity and physical gesture. This distinction will be used throughout the manuscript.

Similar to Neumuth et al. [44], activities are defined as a triple of the used instrument, the performed action and the organ acted on, in this work. For instance, the cutting of the splenic vein with a scalpel is considered an activity. A (surgical) situation is the set of activities which currently occur in the OR. A detailed discussion can be found in chapter 3.3.

Defining the phase is more difficult. There is no consensus in literature apart from the notion that they are higher level descriptions of the current state of the surgery. However, since the purpose of the eventual situation interpretation is to infer which assistance functions should be active at a given moment, phases are defined pragmatically: a phase is a set of situations similar in the medical sense and in need of a common type of assistance, e.g. a specific visualization. Examples of phases in this sense are resections or mobilizations of specific structures.

The possible sequences in which phases can occur chronologically are referred to as surgery plans in this work. The result of the situation interpretation is the recognized phase. Therefore the terms situation interpretation and phase recognition are used anonymously in the following.

3.3. Representation Primitives for Surgical Situations

ORs during a surgery are highly cluttered scenes. To completely describe even snapshots exhaustively, massive amounts of information are necessary. Positions of the surgical staff in the room, device parameters and outputs, position of the patient on the table, vital and anesthesiological parameters, presence of certain instruments are only few examples of salient and noteworthy observations one could use to characterize a situation. All of these are potentially useful in the task of situation interpretation.

However, for practical purposes, it is necessary to restrict the amount of knowledge about the current situation in the OR to reasonable levels. This is not only an issue of processing the data but also of acquiring it. To have arbitrary insight in the current scene, a prohibitive amount of sensors would be necessary. Those sensor would likely interfere with the workflow and increase costs of operation. Therefore it is important to pick a subset of all possible information which is going to be used for the situation interpretation. In other words, the primitives of which the situation model is to be composed of need to be chosen.

Several different approaches have been proposed in the literature to this end. It has been shown that reduction to, for instance, the currently used instrument can suffice to recognize phases during certain interventions [5]. However, it is unlikely that such restrictions generalize well to other types of surgeries. The particular partition into phases and even personal styles of surgeons can lead to several phases employing the same instrument. They, thus, cannot be discriminated based on this feature alone. To avoid workarounds with special and surgery specific features like the inclination of the operating table [53] a more general approach is necessary.

This work focuses on the level of activities (triplets of instrument, action and anatomical structure) to interpret situations. These are the primitives the current situation in the OR of is modeled with. The reasoning for this is that activities are the most fine-grained level of granularity that is symbolic, according to the levels of granularity proposed by Lalys et al. [35]. The lowest level is that of physical gestures. It is concerned with highly specific movement patterns and illuminates more about how actions are performed, than why. The second level of activities on the other hand describes something that usually serves a purpose and has a meaning on its own. Activities are thus the most detailed representation of surgical workflows to posses symbolic and semantic information. As for the practical aspect, it has been shown that such activities can be recognized intraoperatively using advanced image and gesture analysis techniques [52]. An example of a situation in the OR described by the set of the currently occurring activities is shown in Fig. 3.2.

It is important to note however, that limitation to activities is not set in stone. It is a design decision, not a limitation of the knowledge based approach. The use of the ontology allows for extensibility. New concepts and relations can be added to accommodate for new primitives, if they are deemed necessary in the future. For instance, the concept of *surgical action* (sub-classes of which could be *cutting* or *holding*) can be extended with a sister-concept *speech act* (with sub-concepts like *commanding* or *asking*) to include the verbal communication of the surgical staff in the model of the situation. Similarly, other features of interest can be added.

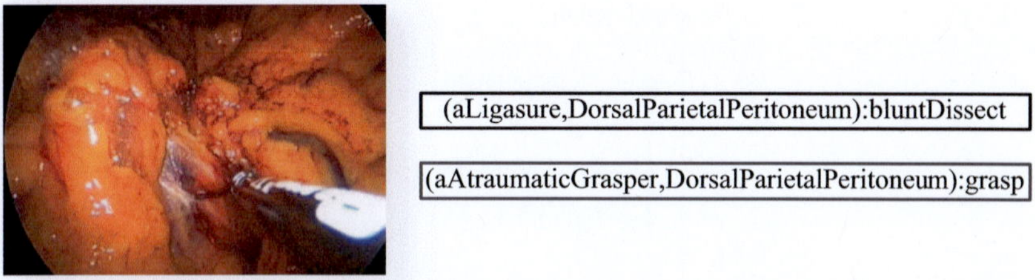

Figure 3.2.: Annotation of a surgical scene with activities

3.4. The Ontology for Laparoscopy

The driving idea behind The Ontology for Laparoscopy is sufficient performance for online, intraoperative reasoning. For this, some aspects of ontological quality and reusability are compromised. Its main advantage is the complete representation of the knowledge in a very concise, resource-conscious way.

To acquire this knowledge the "Teach-Back Method" [34] was used. The idea behind it is as following: First medical experts explain the domain to the engineer, who then in turn teaches the information back, as is it was understood. Possible misunderstandings or missing links can be identified and corrected. This is done to assure mutual understanding.

The ontology was authored with the ontology editor Protege[2]. The concept of the ontology was published in [29]. The individual aspects of The Ontology for Laparascopy are described in the following.

3.4.1. Representation of Formal Knowledge

As elaborated in chapter 3.3, the relevant level of granularity is that of activities. To represent activities, three components are necessary: instruments, actions and anatomical structures.

[2] http://protege.stanford.edu

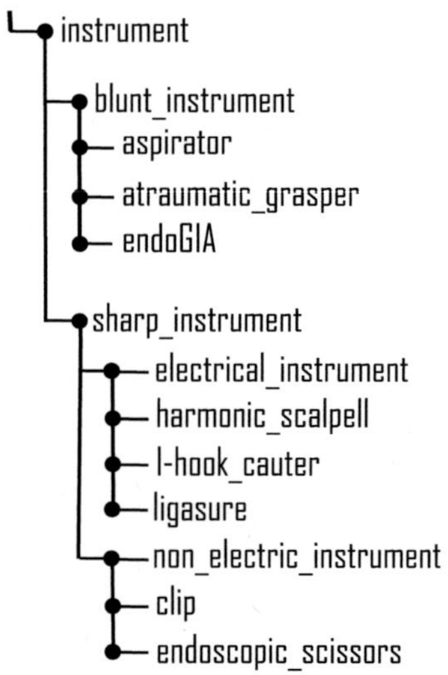

Figure 3.3.: Excerpt of the representation of instruments

Representation of Instruments Instruments are described by TBox concepts. All instruments are sub-concepts of *instrument*. They are categorized according to their properties, such as sharpness or bluntness via appropriate classes which further specialize *instrument*. For instance the l-hook cauter is expressed by *l-hook cauter* $\sqsubseteq$ *electric instrument* $\sqsubseteq$ *sharp instrument* $\sqsubseteq$ *instrument*. An excerpt is shown in Fig. 3.3.

Representation of Actions Actions, like clipping, cutting or grasping, are not described by concepts, but rather by relations. The idea is that an action is a relation between the instrument and the affected anatomical structure. All actions are sub-relations of *surgical action*. They are organized in hierarchical fashion which represents the semantic meaning and groups the individual actions. For instance, *coagulating*, *cutting* and *resecting* are subrelations of *tissue division action*.

Representation of Anatomical Structures Anatomical structures are described similar to instruments. They are also defined as concepts.

Organs are, for instance, all defined as sub-concepts of *organ*. The left renal artery is defined via *left renal artery* $\sqsubseteq$ *artery* $\sqsubseteq$ *vessel* $\sqsubseteq$ *organ*. An excerpt is shown in Fig.3.4.

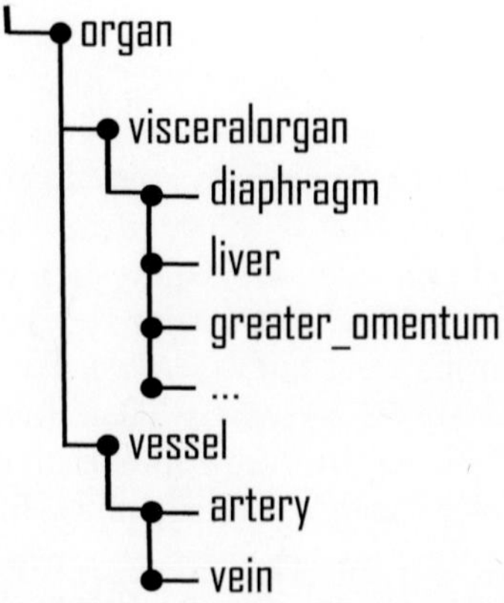

Figure 3.4.: Excerpt of the representation of anatomical structures

The ontology contains 30 relations and 150 concepts with the expressivity of OWL DL. All modeled knowledge is accessible to logical reasoning.

3.4.2. Representation of Experience-based Knowledge

Experience-based knowledge is represented by situations, i.e. the sets of activities currently occurring in the OR. For this, the representations of instruments, actions and anatomical structures need to be combined. This can be done in several ways. In this work two have been chosen for further investigation: the connected and the isolated approach. The difference is that the connected approach connects individual situations and their relation to phases. The isolated approach is concerned with representing just the current situation, with no connection to previous situations or to the level of phases. Both approaches are detailed in the following.

Connected Approach The connected approach aims to represent all activities which occurred during the surgery and the connection to phases.

The phases occurring in the OR are represented as instances of the appropriate classes. Whenever the situation interpretation detects a new phase, an instance of the relation *followed by* is asserted in the ABox between the instances of the newly detected phase and the previous one. This way the temporal order between phases is represented and their occurrence is documented. To indicate that an activity occurred in a certain phase, a relation is asserted between the two instances. However, the ABox formalism can only represent binary relations. To represent that an action belongs to a certain phase, that it affects a certain organ and that it is performed with a certain instruments requires a trinary relation. To work with this limitation of the ABox, actions for the connected approach need to be represented not as relations but as classes. For this, a restructuring of The Ontology of Laprascopy is necessary. Then, the activity is represented by connecting its components with the appropriate relations. The instance of the action class is then connected to the phase instance. This modeling is shown in Fig 3.5. In this way activities, as a whole, can be traced back to their respective phase.

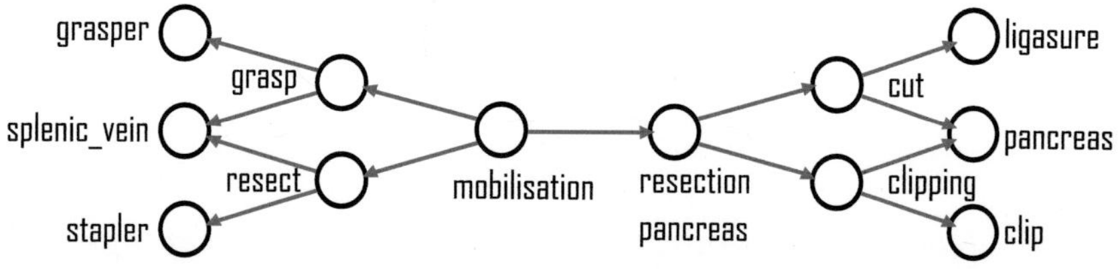

Figure 3.5.: Representation of activities and their connection to phases

Isolated Approach The isolated approach to situation representation restricts the view just on the present, currently occurring events of the surgery. This is valid under the realistic assumption that the current phase can be recognized by looking at just the current activities. In contrast to the connected representation, the detailed representation of past activities can then be omitted. In this case, activities do not need to be explicitly linked to their respective phase. Therefore, only three pieces of information need to be represented to capture the activity.

This opens a new space for simplification of the representation. Binary relation are sufficient to represent an activity in this case. For instance, the occurrence of a scalpel cutting the liver is expressed with the assertions *scaplel(aScalepel) and liver(aLiver) and cutting(aScalpel, aLiver).* Once the activity is over, the assertion is removed from the ABox. Entire situations are then expressed in the ABox as sets of the activities currently in progress. An example is shown in Fig. 3.6.

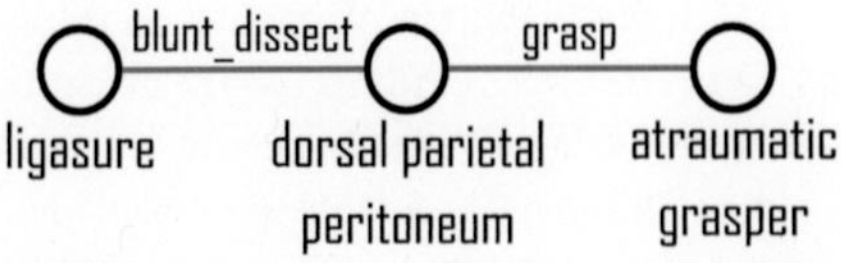

Figure 3.6.: Minimal representation of activities

Comparison of both Approaches The connected representation has the distinct advantage that information about temporal order and the connection of activities to phases is modeled explicitly. Also the entire workflow in modeled. However, precedence information between activities is only preserved at the phase level. The order within a phase is lost. This can be handled either within the interpretation algorithm itself, by adding a new relation representing precedence or time stamps. Both options add complexity though. Furthermore, this solution requires the use of tertary relations, which in turn require workarounds since in OWL only binary relations are allowed.

The isolated method on the other hand, offers a more elegant, simple way of describing the situation. Since only binary relations are used, the resulting expressions are shorter and easier to formulate. Also computation time for reasoning services is reduced. While information about past activities is lost, the history of the surgery is still partly retained in the representation of the surgery plan. Information about which phases already occurred during the intervention is still readily available by separately asserting the *followed by* relation between instances of phase concepts.

Therefore, considering the special emphasis on being light-weight, high-performance, The Ontology for Laparascopy was realized using the isolated approach. While the quality of representation is somewhat compromised, the benefits still outweigh the heavy burden on computation times given by the more complex modeling.

3.4.3. Representation of Surgical Plans

As defined in chapter 3.2, a surgery plan represents all sequences in which phases can occur chronologically. Directed graphs are used as the representational formalism.

Phases are represented by vertices, the precedence relation via edges. This is translated to OWL as follows. Phases are represented as subconcepts of *phase*, another branch of The Ontology for Laprascopy. Their order is defined using the relation *next possible phase* and its inverse *previous phase.* A transition between phases p_1 and p_2 is called valid, if *next possible phase(*p_1*,* p_2*)* is asserted in the ABox. Essentially, *next possible phase(*p_1 *,* p_2*)* represents the knowledge, that p_2 be a follow-up to p_1. The surgery plan is implemented by creating instances of all phases of the surgery in the ABox and and all connections with the *next possible phase* relation. An example is shown in Fig. 3.7.

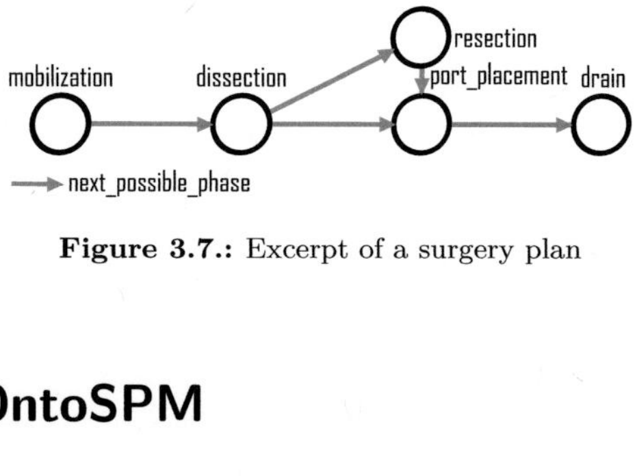

Figure 3.7.: Excerpt of a surgery plan

3.5. LapOntoSPM

The approach to knowledge representation in the previous section contains all the vocabulary necessary to describe laparascopic interventions at the considered granularity levels. Emphasis is put on a simple, minimalist representation to keep reasoning time low. However, requirements on quality and ease of sharing had to be sacrificed. LapOntoSPM, on the other hand, focuses on just these points.

The best way to ensure reusabilty is to reuse other established ontologies as much as possible. This way, there is, by design, a great overlap in terminology with other ontologies. As an added benefit, the quality of the representation tends to improve, if established ontologies of a high quality standard are used. Therefore the work is integrated into OntoSPM, a core ontology for surgical process models [13].

In the domain of surgical process modeling, OntoSPM, is beginning to emerge as a new standard. Although still in its infancy, at the time this work has been done, it is already a high quality ontology for its domain. Furthermore, due to the early cycle in its development, it was possible to collaborate with the initiators of OntoSPM to not only work on LapOntoSPM, but also on OntoSPM.

OntoSPM itself is based on BFO[3](Basic Formal Ontology). BFO is an upper-level ontology which provides highly abstract classes. They are specified to less abstract concepts for the description of general surgical processes in OntoSPM. The idea is to further specialize OntoSPM in so called application ontologies for specific purposes.

LapOntoSPM is a specialization of OntoSPM for laparoscopic surgeries. The use of OntoSPM as a core ontology not only adds restrictions which facilitate quality but also ensures compatibility with other ontologies built with OntoSPM or BFO.

To further ensure reusability a number of highly prominent ontologies have been imported. This increases overlap with existing ontologies. Specifically LapOntoSPM includes parts of the Foundational Model of Anatomy(FMA) [47], the Information Artefact Ontology (IAO) [4] and Unit Ontology (UO) [5]. An illustration of the relations between the ontologies is shown in Fig. 3.8. The FMA is a widely used ontology for anatomical knowledge. The IAO is used to describe numerical measurements of distances and mass relevant for the surgical domain. UO is used to specify units in which measurement values are quantified. The modeling in LapOntoSPM is detailed in the following section. LapOntoSPM was published in [21].

[3] http://ifomis.uni-saarland.de/bfo/
[4] http://purl.obolibrary.org/obo/iao
[5] https://code.google.com/p/unit-ontology/

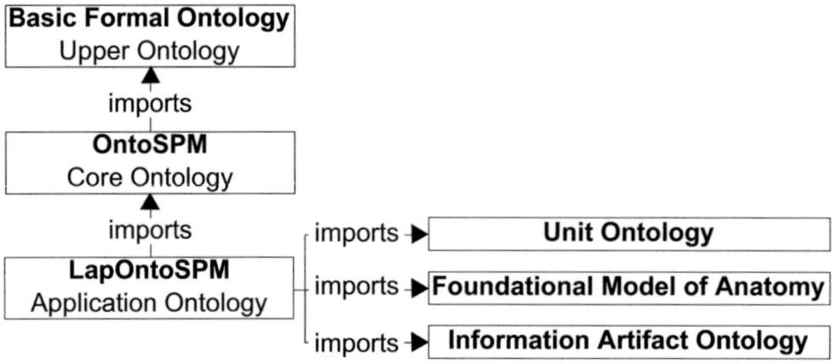

Figure 3.8.: Relationships between the different ontolgies

3.5.1. Representation of Formal Knowledge

As in chapter 3.4.1 about The Ontology for Laparascopy, instruments, actions and anatomical structures need to be described with LapOntoSPM. In contrast to The Ontology for Laparascopy, more emphasis is placed on quality and integration into existing ontologies. Therefore the modeling is more complicated, but also has higher semantic content.

Representation of Instruments To model information about instruments, OntoSPM offers the class *surgical instrument* $\sqsubseteq$ *medical device* $\sqsubseteq$ *physical object* $\sqsubseteq$ *object*. Further specialization takes place in the application ontology. For the task of context-awareness and analysis of surgical workflows, the instrument function, i.e. the set of actions the instrument is intended to perform, is very important. Therefore these functions are part of the model and used as the main categorization criterion.

Functions, in the BFO sense of the concept *function*, are elucidated as dispositions which exist due to the physical make-up of the considered object. Intentional design is also explicitly entailed. For this purpose the concept *function of instrument* $\sqsubseteq$ *function* is used as the upper class for all instrument functions (e.g. *to cut* or *to coagulate*).

Instrument and their functions are related via the *has instrument function* relation. This is declared to be a sub-relation of the BFO relation *has function*. For example the class *endoscopic scissors* is declared subclass of *has instrument function some to cut*, representing that endoscopic scissors have the function to cut. Multiple functions are modeled by adding several such statements. This is used to further group instruments. Equivalence concepts such as *cutting instrument* or *grapsing instrument* cover instruments having that particular function. Those are further grouped, for instance to *tissue division instrument* which is the union of *coagulating instrument*, *cutting instrument* and *dissecting instrument*. Instruments are automatically classified by reasoning over the TBox.

This categorization of instruments is not restricting. Other features, such as form, can still be included later on, for instance to support shape-based recognition of instruments. Since multiple inheritance is allowed in OWL, concepts can have an arbitrary number of super-concepts and thus can be part of several hierarchies simultaneously. The addition of more information and structure leaves the categorization by function intact.

Representation of Actions Actions are represented by the concept *action* $\sqsubseteq$ *process* in OntoSPM. The appropriate actions for laprascopy (e.g. *coagulating*) are added as sub-concepts here. They are further described by the integration in the inheritance structure of OntoSPM, which categorizes actions into groups (*holding an object*, *dissecting an object...*). In this way, semantic information about the actions is represented.

Instrument functions and actions are also connected. The concept function in BFO is declared as *function* $\sqsubseteq$ *disposition* $\sqsubseteq$ *realizable entity*. Realizable entities can be understood as attributes or features of things which are realized in a process. An example of this is the tendency of blood to coagulate. The coagulation in an inherent property of the blood yet it needs a process (of bleeding/being exposed to air) to come to fruition. Similarly, the genetic predisposition of a person to get cancer is inherent to the person, yet needs a process (that of living/being alive) to materialize. The functions of an instrument is also realized in a process. For instance, the function *to cut* of *endoscopic scissors* is realized by the action *cutting*. Consequently,instrument functions and actions are connected via the BFO relation *realized in*, e.g. *to cut is realized in some cutting*.

Representation of Anatomical Structures Anatomical structures in LapOntoSPM are represented using a subset of the FMA ontology. The

FMA is used by numerous ontologies and thus contributes to reusability. The reason for reusing just a subset is that the FMA contains far too many concepts which are irrelevant to laparascopic surgery to warrant a complete import. Only selected structures are reused. The extraction was done using OntoFox [63], a web-based ontology extraction service.

The relationships between anatomical structures, instruments and actions are summarized in Fig.3.9. Instruments have functions, realized by actions. Actions affect anatomical structures and use instruments to do so.

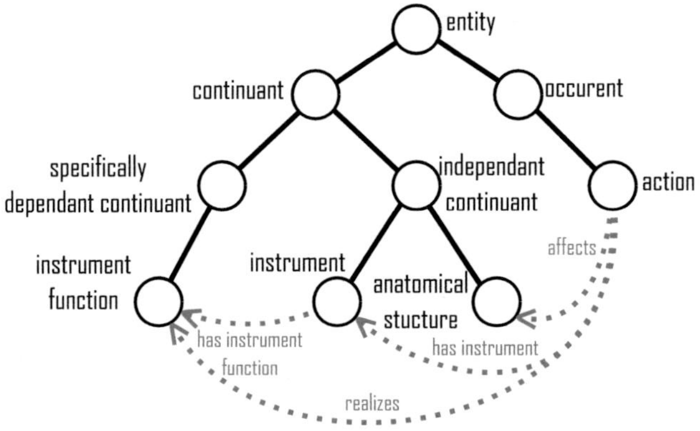

Figure 3.9.: Relationships between anatomical structures, instruments and actions

Representation of Measurements Additionally to instruments, actions and anatomical structures, measurements of lengths and mass can be very important during laparoscopic interventions. For instance, it might be relevant to represent lengths of resection margins or incisions. Similarly blood loss or the amount of injected substances oftentimes needs to be expressed numerically. For this purpose, a subset of the Information Artifact Ontology is used. The extraction was again done using OntoFox. The idea is to describe length and mass as qualities, dependent on some bearer. The measurements are then attached to qualities with labels denominating the measurement value and its unit. The unit are integrated via the Unit Ontology.

Specifically, the idea in the Information Artifact Ontology is to separate measurements from the quality being measured. The reasoning is that measurements are often noisy, in some cases inevitably so. Consequently, several measurement of the same quality with different values can coexist simultaneously. Therefore, they should be explicitly represented as what they are: measurements, and not as values of the quality. Measurements are represented as instances of *quality measurement* connected to the quality via the *is quality measurement of* relation. They are defined by a *unit label*, connected via *has measurement unit label* and a data property *has measurement value*. An illustation is shown in Fig. 3.10.

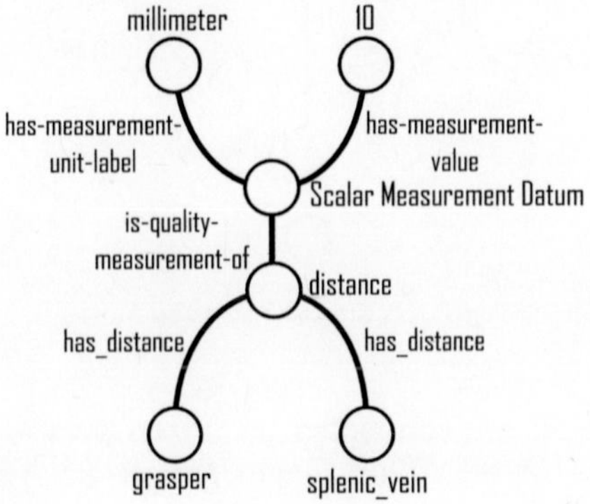

Figure 3.10.: Measurement of distance between a grasper and a splenic vein

3.5.2. Representation of Experience-based Knowledge

The aim of the representation of the surgical workflow is to represent the occurrences in the OR in a formal model. In the case considered in this work, this entails all activities that were performed during the surgery and their connection to phases and surgeries. In contrast to the representation with The Ontology for Laparascopy, LapOntoSPM represents the entire workflow, instead of just individual, situational snapshots.

In OntoSPM, the levels of granularity, i.e. surgical procedure, phase, stage, step and action, are defined as sub-classes of the BFO concept *process*, which is a sub-class of *occurant*. The concepts at the lower end of the

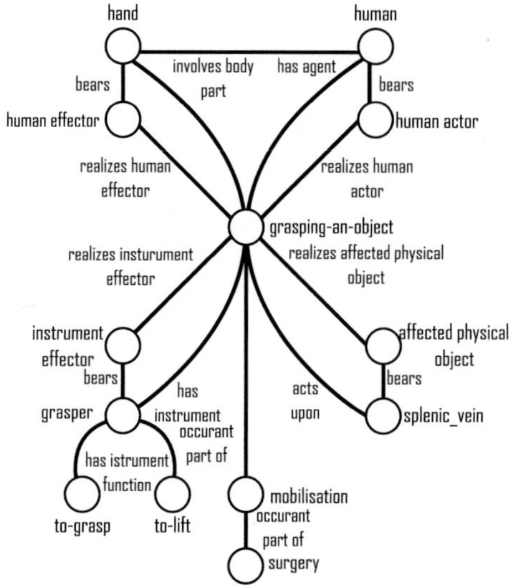

Figure 3.11.: Excerpt of a Surgical Process Model in LapOntoSPM

granularity spectrum are connected using the *part of occurant* relation or a specialization thereof. That means actions are part of a phase and phases are parts of a surgery and so on.

The representation at the level of activities is as follow: actions are represented as instances of the appropriate type. They are connected to the instrument that is being used via the *has instrument* relation and to the affected anatomical structure via *acts upon*. Apart from that, some additional information is modeled. The surgeon himself, represented as an instance of *human*, is declared as the performer of the action with an assertion of the relation *has agent*. Similarly, the hand being used is represented with another instance and the relation *involves body part* to the corresponding action. The roles of *human effector*, *human actor*, *instrument effector* and *affected physical object* are realized by the actions, as denoted with the appropriate relations. By adding new activities, a complete and semantically rich surgical process model is created. As an example, the representation of a grasper grasping a splenic vein is illustrated in Fig.3.11.

3.5.3. Representation of Surgical Plans

The surgical plan describes constraints on the temporal order in which phases can occur during the surgery. Informally, they can be described using directed graphs. For this purpose, the relation *next possible phase* and its inverse *previous phase* are used. This is similar to the way it is done in The Ontology for Laparascopy, as described in chapter 3.4.1.

3.6. Summary

In this chapter, two ontologies which offer a foundation of formal knowledge to be used to interpret situations are presented: The Ontology for Laparascopy and LapOntoSPM. The ontologies offer a language for the formalization of experience-based knowledge, as seen in chapter 3.4.2 and 3.5.2, which is connected with formal knowledge.

Apart from requirements on content, other factors were taken into account when designing the ontologies. Particularly, it is important to consider the issue of reuse. This entails both the reuse of other, established ontologies as well as making the ontology accessible by others. The use-case of intraoperative context-awareness however, imposes restrictions on the run-time. This is in conflict with the other requirements as a problem specific, reduced ontology is more likely to be more computationally lightweight.

Two different ontologies were developed. The Ontology for Laparascopy is application focused. It does not make use of upper ontologies. No existing ontologies are reused. This approach has the advantage of expressing situations with a very small amount of instances. Computation times are short. Yet, the knowledge represented is limited. For instance, there is no information about roles or people involved in the procedure. This is of lesser importance for context-awareness, but crucial for other applications. While a great solution for the problem of context-awareness, it is difficult to reuse and share the represented knowledge.

LapOntoSPM counters this problem. It is integrated into OntoSPM, a developing standard for the representation of surgical process models under the upper-ontology BFO. Also other ontologies (namely the Information

Artifact Ontology, the Foundational Model of Anatomy and the Unit Ontology) are reused. This greatly facilitates integration and interoperability with other ontolgies. Due to the strong focus on reuse of established ontologies the quality of the ontology is increased.

LapOntoSPM and The Ontology for Laprascopy are not independent. They are connected at the lowest level of the inheritance hierarchy with the *same as* relation. That means that for instance, concepts like *scalpel* are considered the same. In this way, The Ontology for Laprascopy can benefit from LapOntoSPM, if necessary.

Thus it is shown that formal medical knowledge can be formalized in a reusable, generic way. The representation can be used to describe surgical situations and entire workflows and thus represent experience-based knowledge that is linked to the formal knowledge.

4. Situation Interpretation with Formal Knowledge

Rule-based systems using formal knowledge have been traditionally used in Artificial Intelligence to model human cognition. It fact, people often tend to naturally express knowledge in the form of "if-then" rules. It also explains at least parts of human cognition [51].

Especially for situation interpretation, rules have several benefits. They are readable by man and machine alike. This makes verification and checking by medical experts rather easy. It also allows automatic consistency checking. This does not only benefit the safety aspect but also helps build trust among surgeons. It allows deep insight in the inner workings of the system, unlike machine-learning-based black boxes. Furthermore, in medicine, there are huge amounts of knowledge available from literature and experts alike. In a way, it is wasteful to discard this formal knowledge and rely only on machine learning to learn what medical experts already know. This is especially important in the considered domain, as annotation of surgical workflow is very resource intensive.

Despite these benefits, there is little use of formal knowledge and rules in the current state of the art for situation interpretation, as shown in chapter 2. Thus the motivation for this work. The goal is to allow recognition of surgical phases without any training samples.

The core idea of the proposed approach is to extract knowledge systematically from experts to define conditions which indicate a transition from one phase to another. These conditions and a method to extract the knowledge are detailed in 4.1.

To formalize the rules, an appropriate rule language needs to be chosen. At best, it should be **non-proprietary**, well **supported by tools** and

expressive enough to elegantly represent the rules and make them **easy to share**. This helps avoid limited solutions which are tied to the current application and software environment.

The rest of the chapter is concerned with the implementation of this idea with different rule languages. Specifically, nRQL (new Racer Query Language) [14], ad-hoc rules with OWL API (Web Ontology Language Application Programming Interface) [15], SWRL (Semantic Web Rule Language) [46] and SQWRL (Semantic Query-Enhanced Web Rule Language) [45] are investigated. The general idea that is expressed in these representational formalism is explained in the following section.

4.1. Concept for Formal Knowledge-based Situation Interpretation

The idea behind the approach is to create "if-then" rules for each phase. If a condition of a rule, for instance the presence of a certain activity, is fulfilled, the corresponding phase is considered to be currently occurring in the OR. This interpretation cycle, i.e. the checking of the if-conditions of each rule happens every time the model of the situation changes. That is the case at each beginning and end of an activity.

The conditions considered are:

- **Validness** The Validness refers to whether there is a valid transition between one phase to another. A transition is called valid if it does not contradict the surgery plan.
- **Phase Specificness** The Phase Specificness refers to whether there is an activity in the current model which is strongly connected to and indicative of the beginning of a specific phase. Such activities are called Triggering Activities.

If both conditions apply, i.e. if it is possible to transition from phase a to phase b and a Triggering Activity for b has been observed, a transition to phase b is assumed. Alternatively, only the Phase Specificness can be used, if the surgery plan is be ignored or cannot be formulated.

Extracting the formal knowledge for Validness and Phase Specificness from experts is difficult, especially concerning tacit knowledge. It is therefore vital to have a methodical, structured approach. In this case, the so called "Teach-Back Method" was used [34]. The basic idea behind this approach is to let the domain expert, i.e. the surgeon explain the performance of the surgery and the relations between activities and phases to the knowledge engineer. In the second step the knowledge engineer reiterates the information, i.e. teaches it back to the surgeon. During this process the surgeon can identify any gaps or misunderstandings and correct them. Possible misconceptions can be cleared up and eventually mutual understanding is assured.

Another advantage of this approach is that the Teach-Back Method is commonly used in medical health care to ensure informed patient consent. Therefore it is already established in the medical community. It is known and trusted among clinical staff.

4.2. Realization with nRQL

nRQL (new Racer Query Language) is a query language for RacerPro [14], a reasoner for DL. It can be used to query ABoxes as well as TBoxes. Apart from conjunctive rules, nRQL allows complex queries with constructors like union as well as Negation as failure (NAF) and other highly expressive constructs. The work with nRQL was published in [24].

As evident from its name, nRQL is meant to issue queries. To express rules, the idea is to formulate a query which asks for individuals satisfying the Validness or Phase Specificness condition. If the query returns an empty set, the condition is not satisfied. Otherwise the phase is assumed to be currently occurring.

To express queries, nRQL works with variables, which refer to individuals of the ABox. A variable is bound to an individual if this individual satisfies the query. Satisfies means that the statement resulting from substituting all variables with the individuals they are bound to holds in the current situation. A variable x which can be bound to individuals of the concepts C is declared by *(C ?x)*. For instance, in nRQL syntax, the query *(retrieve (?x) (liver ?x))*

retrieves all individuals that can be bound to the variable x. That corresponds to all individuals which can be substituted for x to make the expression *(liver ?x)* true. In simple terms: the query retrieves all individuals of the concept *liver*.

nRQL also allows for conjunction. To retrieve all diseased livers, i.e. all individuals of the concept *liver* and *diseased structure*, the following term can be used:

(retrieve (?x) (and (liver ?x) (diseased structure?x))

Relations, too, can be used in these expressions via *(r ?x ?y)*. In this case the relation r needs to hold between individuals that can be bound to x and y.

This is sufficient to formulate Validness and Phase Specificness. The set of phases which can be transitioned to from the phase *mobilization* is retrieved by:

(retrieve (?p) (and (phase ?p)
(mobilization ?m)) (next possible phase ?m ?p))

Triggering Activities can also be expressed. For instance, this query checks for risk situation where a sharp instrument is near a vital structure:

(retrieve (and (sharp instrument ?inst) (vital structure ?c)) (near ?x ?y))

To check for both Validness and Phase Specificity, a conjunction is used.

In these examples, the modeling of The Ontology of Laparascopy has been used. The formulation of the rules for LapOntoSPM is analogous, yet more verbose since the action are described as concepts, which adds more variables and makes the rules more difficult to read.

nRQL is certainly expressive enough to formulate the necessary rules. However, it is a proprietary language bound to a specific reasoner, namely RacerPro. It therefore is limited to a small set of available tools.

4.3. Realization with OWL API

The OWL API offers powerful capabilities for creating, manipulating and serializing OWL Ontologies [15]. It grants unified access to reasoning facilities of popular and well established reasoners such as FaCT++ [58], HermiT [48] and Pellet [49]. OWL API allows to query contents of the ABox and TBox in a programmatic way, which allows their processing in the supported programming language. In this work the Java implementation of OWL API is used. This allows very expressive and profound manipulation and analysis of the model, given the possibilities of a Turing-complete language. The work on this was published in [30].

The rules can then be implemented by using OWL API to query for contents of the ABOX, whereby OWL reasoning facilities can be used.

However this comes with a significant drawback. While the formulation of rules is flexible, the rules are still partly formulated in an all-purpose language. This makes verification, sharing and standardization difficult and does not fit well into the overall OWL tool-chain. The extended expressiveness, given by the Turing-complete language, is only be of use if more complex models of the surgery plan are used.

4.4. Realization with SWRL

The Semantic Web Rule Language (SWRL) is a standard rule language for OWL [46]. It allows the formulation of Horn-like rules. The work with SWRL has been published in [28].

The rules are defined by an antecedent (body) and consequent (head). Syntactically, body and head are separated by $\Rightarrow$. If the condition of the body is fulfilled, the contents of the head are asserted in the ABox. Similarly to nRQL, it works with variables. For instance the fact that the liver is a vital organ is asserted by this rule:

$$\textit{liver(?x)} \Rightarrow \textit{vital structure(?x)}$$

In this case *liver(?x)* is the body, *vital structure(?x))* is the head. The rule states that all individuals that are of the concept *liver* are necessarily also individuals of the concept *vital structure.*

The following is restricted to the presentation of the formulation of the body. The formulation of the head is explained afterwards. The Validness can be expressed as part of the body using conjunction via *and* in SWRL:

phase(?p) and current phase(?current) and
next possible phase(?current, ?p)

Intuitively, the variable p refers to an instance of *phase* and *current* to an instance of *current phase.* Furthermore, the relation *next possible phase* must be asserted between them. Put differently, p refers to all phases for which the validness condition is fulfilled. Phase Specificness can be formulated similarly. In the case of the phase of port placement in a pancreatic resection, this would be:

port(?instrument) and Abdomen(?structure) and
place(?instrument, ?structure)

In other words, it is checked whether there are instances *instrument* of *port* being placed on an *abdomen.* This is the generally applicable template for the creation of SWRL rules. If both Validness and Phase Specificity are to be considered, the conjunction of both expressions is used.

The formulation of the head is not straightforward. One would assume that it can just be set to *current phase(?p).* However this is not the case due to expressiveness limitation of SWRL. Particularly, the monotonicity requires that new, additional information does not invalidate previous reasoning results. In this particular case, this implies that once a phase has been declared a *current phase*, no SWRL rules can change that. Outside intervention is necessary to solve this problem. This makes it difficult to just set the head to *current phase(?p).* To work around this limitation, the head of the rules is set to *detected phase(?p).* After each interpretation cycle the ABox is cleaned up using an external program. If a *detected phase* is asserted, the outside program removes the assertion *current phase* of the current phase and marks it as a *visited phase* to signify its occurrence. Then, the newly detected phase is asserted to be no longer a *detected phase* but of type *current phase*. After this setup, all phases of type *current phase* are regarded as the result of the interpretation. In the beginning, *start* is declared a *current phase* to initialize the system. This concepts is illustrated in Fig.4.1.

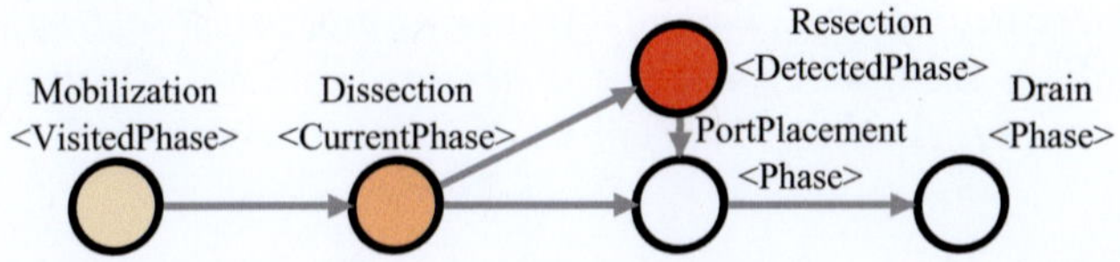

Figure 4.1.: Visited, current and detected phases as part of the surgery plan

SWRL offers a standardized way of implementing rules, and has a solid amount of tools available. Specifically, it is supported by OWL API and several reasoners like Hermit and Pellet. It has also a well-defined semantics and allows for a clear, human readable representation. While the use of SWRL is a very feasible approach to situation interpretation, there are drawbacks. Particularly the monotonicity of the SWRL rules forces outside retraction of previous assertions. Both are practices that are best to avoid. Furthermore, it adds otherwise unnecessary overhead to the interpretation algorithm regarding the management of the retraction. When only considering the current situation, these drawbacks are not too damaging. Yet when considering the entire surgical process model, other means of rule formulation should be considered.

4.5. Realization with SQWRL

SQWRL is a SWRL-based language which adds the ability to issue queries to OWL ontologies, see [21].

The idea behind the SQWRL-approach is to implement the "rules as queries" idea from the nRQL approach with SWRL. Queries are issued to determine Validness and Phase Specificity by looking for the empty set as a result. Conceptually this is as described in chapter 4.2 for nRQL.

For this purpose the body of the SWRL-rules is used as the query. This can be easily done as SQWRL can be understood as an extension of SWRL. Instead of making assertions about the individuals that satisfy the condition in the body, they are just returned as the result of the query. An example of a SQWRL query for a modeling in LapOntoSPM is:

port(?instrument) and Abdomen(?structure) and place(?action) and acts upon(?action, ?structure) and has instrument(?action, ?instrument) $\Rightarrow$ *sqwrl:select(?instrument. ?action, ?structure)*

In this example the similarity with SWRL is obvious. The set of activities is queried with a port being placed on the abdomen. If the set is not empty this Triggering Activity is detected.

This example applies to a modeling with LapOntoSPM. The modeling with The Ontology for Laparascopy is analogous. SQWRL is thus expressive enough and it is non-proprietary. However, not all tools support this extension of SWRL yet. This affects sharing of knowledge, but its syntactic and semantic proximity to SWRL lesser this problem to some extent.

4.6. Evaluation

The purpose of this evaluation is to quantify the ability of the formal approach to recognize phases. The algorithm is evaluated on manually labeled annotations of actual surgeries. This approach has several benefits. Apart from the reproducability of results, the problem of using the system intraoperatively while maintaining medical relevance and a firm grounding in the actual processes in the OR is avoided. Note that the choice of the rule language does not change the meaning of the rules. Only the syntax changes. The rules still capture the same Validness and Phase Specificity, no matter in which language they are expressed. However, there can be differences in run-time.

The evaluation is performed both with the Ontology for Laparascopy and LapOntoSPM, using SWRL and SQWRL respectively.

To show that the algorithm is able to generalize over several surgery types, pancreatic resections and adrenalectomies are considered. Furthermore, distorted versions of the annotations are used to evaluate robustness. In actual, real-word application the data is likely to be distorted in some way, too. For this purposes, a method to systematically add noise to evaluation data was developed.

4.6.1. Evaluation Method

The following describes how the annotation were obtained and distorted to simulate sensor noise. Then the quality measures are introduced. Afterwards the results of the evaluation are presented and discussed.

Acquisition of Annotated Surgeries

For the acquisition of annotated surgeries, 11 pancreatic resections and 5 adrenalectomies have been recorded. Specifically, the output of the endoscope has been stored as video footage. For the annotation, the SwanSuite [43] was used. It is a a commercially available software package for recording workflows. Although not limited in scope, it is specifically geared to the annotation of medical processes and therefore a great fit for the application at hand. An exemplary excerpt is shown in Fig.4.2.

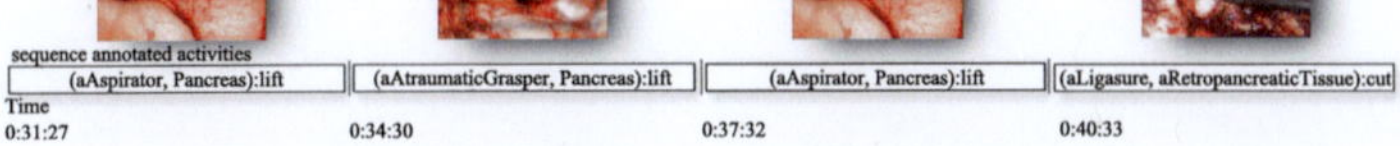

Figure 4.2.: Example of an annotation

Each annotation consists of a list of activities, i.e. tupels of the surgical instrument, action and the anatomical structure acted upon, along with a time stamp denoting begin and end of the activity (which is equivalent to the ones of the action). With clinical partners the surgery types were partitioned in phases. They are described in Fig.4.1 and in Fig.4.2. The relevant statistics about the annotations are shown in Table 4.3.

Phase of pancreasresection	Description
Port Placement	Insertion of surgical instruments and endoscope
Mobilization	Transsection of the gastrocolic ligament
Dissection	Dissection of the parietal peritoneum
Resection	Removal of pathologic pancreas tissue
Closure	Removal of resected tissue in a specimen bag
Drain	Drainage in case of pancreatic fistula or bleeding

Table 4.1.: Phases of the pancreas resection.

Phase of Adrenalectomy	Description
Port Placement	Insertion of surgical instruments and endoscope
Mobilization	Mobilization of adjacent adhesions and the colon to access gerota's fascia
Dissection	Cutting of gerota's fascia to access the adrenal gland
Resection	Resection of the adrenal gland
Closure	Removal of the adrenal gland in a specimen bag
Drain	Drainage in case of bleeding

Table 4.2.: Phases of the adrenalectomy.

	average number of activities	average number of phases	average duration
Pancreasresection	501	12	90 min
Adrenalectomy	221	9	49 min

Table 4.3.: Average number of activities, phases and duration of annotated surgeries.

Addition of noise to Annotated Surgeries

Since the annotations are purely symbolical, the best way to distort them is not obvious. For this evaluation, noise is added in a controlled fashion. Several levels of noise are introduced. They signify how strongly that data is changed from the original. Specifically, it determinates the percentage of activities which are altered. To systematically cover a wider range of distortion, six levels are used: 0%, 10%, 20%, 30%, 40% and 50%.

The next problem is to determine how to apply the distortion to an activity. To arrive at distorted yet still plausible activities, the ontology is used. Each activity is distorted by randomly selecting a component of each activity (i.e. instrument, action or structure). This is then exchanged with a randomly chosen subclass of the appropriate ontological concept. This way it is guaranteed, that for instance instruments will only be changed to other instruments and action will only replace other actions. This is illustrated in Fig.4.3.

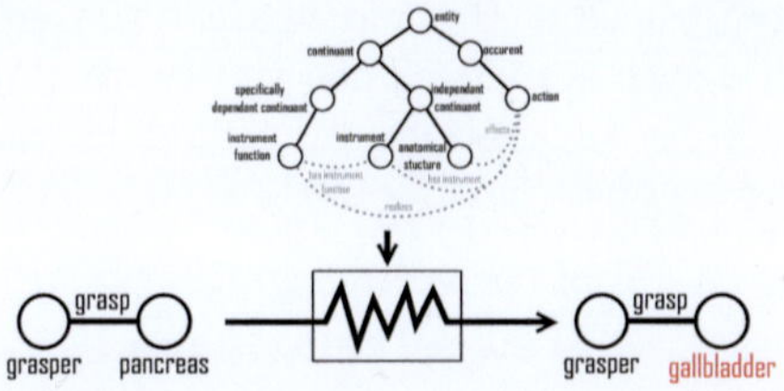

Figure 4.3.: Distorting activities by exchanging components using the ontology

The phases are not distorted, as they represent the ground truth against which the algorithm is measured. During the evaluation, this data is not accessible to the algorithm and only used to determine quality.

Quality Measures for Phase Recognition

There are several ways to quantify the quality of interpretation algorithms. Currently, there is no agreement in the community about how results should be reported and methods vary between publications.

The proposed quality measure is to fulfill several requirements. For once, it needs to be a realistic representation of the expected performance of the system in intraoperative use. That is, it needs to measure how well the visualizations are going to fit the situation in actual use. Secondly, the quality measure needs to provide better insight about which errors are made. Particularly it is interesting to see how well the algorithm can distinguish between given phase, i.e. how likely it is to confuse a certain phase with another. Thirdly, the algorithm needs to be stable, in the sense that the recognition rate does not fluctuate widely in different executions when given the same data. Lastly, the quality measure must consider timing since the recognition has real-time constraints.

In this thesis the following quality measures are considered: recognition rate, confusion matrix, variance and run-time. They quality measures are explained below.

Recognition Rate The Overall Recognition Rate is determined as follows: first, the recognized phase is checked against the ground truth at the beginning and end of each activity. Then the eventual results is computed as the fraction of correct recognitions and overall checks made. That is:

$$\frac{\#\text{ of correct recognitions}}{\#\text{ of overall recognitions}}$$

This allows for a quick and easily reproducible quality assessment, independent of run-time characteristics and hardware setups. This measure also has a great practical value. It is an estimate of the percentage of time the correct phase is found and thus the percentage of time the right visualization is displayed.

Confusion Matrix The recognition rates consider only overall performance. However, oftentimes a more detailed look on the characteristics is desired. Specifically, it is often of interest which phases are recognized well and which ones are not. Moreover, insight which phases tend to get confused with others is important to better asses the algorithms.

For this purpose, confusion matrices are a perfect solution. Each element of the matrix encodes the number of times the phase in the row was recognized as the one in the column. Incidentally, the diagonal entries represent the number of correct recognitions. Confusion matrices are color coded. White denotes the minimal value and black shows the highest. Such representations are more intuitive and easier to grasp visually.

Variance The formal approach is clearly deterministic. If given the same input data, it will always yield the same results. Yet, since distorted data is used, it is not guaranteed that for the same level of noise, there will always be the same recognition rate. It can fluctuate depending on which activities are distorted and which remain intact. The evaluation is therefore performed 10 times on each samples. This data is used to compute the Recognition Rate as average over all iterations and also to compute the variance to quantify the fluctuation.

Run-Time As the eventual system is to run intraopeartively, real-time constraints need to be taken into account. Therefore the average time it takes to recognize the phase is measured. This quantifies the delay between a situation interpretation being triggered and the recognized phase being available to adapt the assistance system.

4.6.2. Results and Discussion

To perform the evaluation, Triggering Activities were extracted using the teach-back method. This resulted in a formalization of the surgery types. The phases considered are explained in Fig.A.1, Fig.A.4 and Fig.A.7, the Triggering activities in Fig.A.2, Fig.A.5 and Fig.A.8. Eventually, the surgery plan was created, as shown in Fig.A.3, Fig.A.6 and Fig.A.9.

The recognition rates for the formal approach are shown in Fig. 4.4 for pancreas resection and adrenalectomy. As is evident, the algorithm performs very well in the undistorted case. However, the performance deteriorates quickly, when noise is introduced.

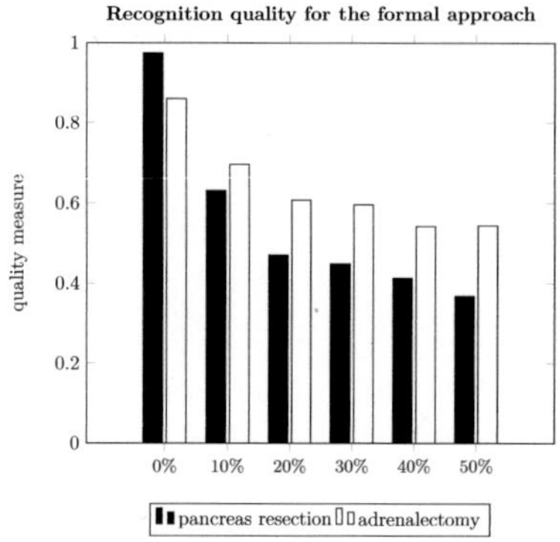

Figure 4.4.: Quality measure at varying distortion levels

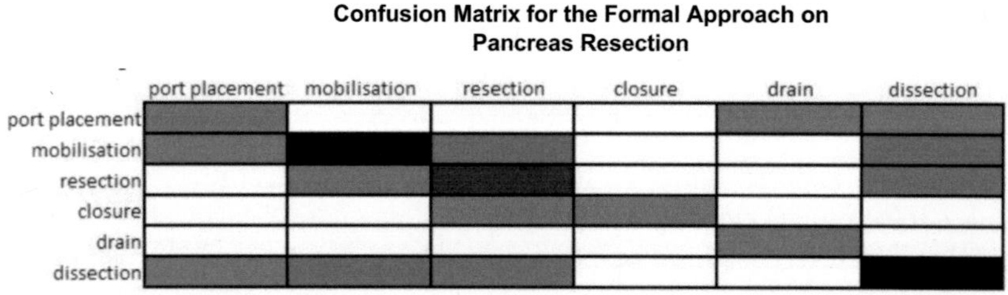

Figure 4.5.: Confusion Matrix showing which phases got confused. Darker values signify higher incidents.

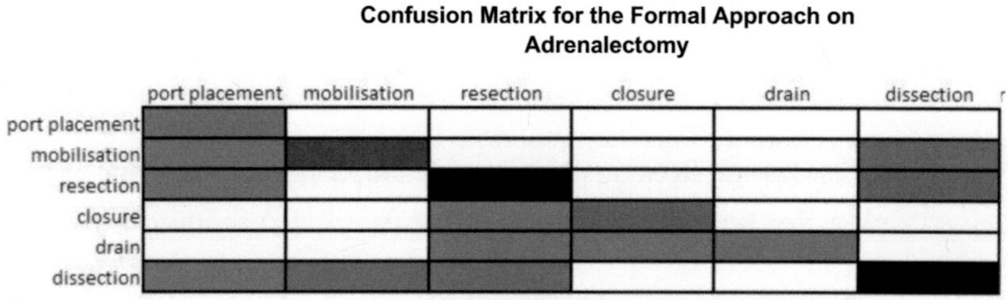

Figure 4.6.: Confusion Matrix showing which phases got confused. Darker values signify higher incidents.

The confusion matrices are shown in Fig. 4.5 for the pancreas resection and in Fig.4.6 for adrenalectomy. As is evident, all phase can be recognized. The vast majority of mobilization, resection and dissection are recognized correctly. However there are false recognitions. Phases which are close to one another in time, like port placement and mobilization can be confused at some points. Also errors occur when an interrupted phase is resumed. For example, after the placement of a port and the recognition the port placement, the algorithm waits for a Triggering Activity to fall back to the previous phase. However, this is usually not instantaneous. Sometimes the Triggering Activities are just not specific enough, i.e. occur in several phases or there are transitions which violate the surgery plan. Yet for the most part, as shown by the recognition rates, the correct phase is found.

The algorithm proved to be quite stable. The variance, i.e. the measure of fluctuation of the recognition rate due to different outcomes of the distortion process vary from 0 for the undistorted case to a maximum of 0.037. The variance of 0 in the undistorted case is not surprising, since the algorithm is deterministic and the input does not change. Therefore, the same results are obtained every time, without any fluctuation.

The evaluation was performed with the Ontology for Laparascopy with SWRL rules and LapOntoSPM with SQWRL. There was no difference in recognition quality. However run-time per recognition increased from 0.5s to 1.8s when using LapOntoSPM.

The results prove that rule-based situation interpretation is fit to provide context-awareness in complex, realistic and medically relevant scenarios.

The recognition quality is high with undistorted data, yet degenerates quickly when noise is added. The rules do have a certain kind of ability to overcome noise. For once, only noise that affects Triggering Activities has an effect on the recognition rate. Even when Triggering Activities are affected, i.e. Triggering Activities are not recognized as such or non-Triggering Activities are changed to appear so, the system can still yield correct answers. For instance, if the concept *cutting instrument* is used in a rule, then all distortions which change the instrument to something that is still a *cutting instrument*, will not affect that rule. However, if some completely different instrument is substituted, the rule will have problems. This is especially important in case of the treated structure. The rules are quite strict in that case.

As for the run-time, the system works quick enough for real-time application. A recognition cycle with SWRL and The Ontology for Laparacopy takes 0.5s. This number increases to 1.8s with LapOntoSPM and SQWRL. This is mainly due to two factors. The richer representation of the workflow leads to a greater number of individuals in the ABox, increasing reasoning time. The other reason for increased run times is more technical. Since SQWRL is not supported by many reasoners yet, ABox contents need to be copied between two reasoners to enable all required reasoning services. The copying and redundant processing heavily increases run time.

Despite the increased run-time, the approach with LapOntoSPM is still valuable. For once, as reasoners mature, support for SQWRL and similar standards will likely increase and make time consuming synchronization between reasoners obsolete. This development alone is sufficient for real-time performance. Even without such advancements, with a recognition duration of fewer than two seconds, the system is usable. In practical application, it means that the recognition and thus the adaption of assistance functions will be delayed for less than two seconds. In most practical scenarios this is good enough. The problem can also easily be tackled with more powerful hardware, since the evaluation was performed on a simple laptop computer. Additionally, it is possible to extract subsets of the ontology and use limited and less computationally demanding variations of LapOntoSPM if performance is critical and the additional semantic content is not needed. Overall, the increase of computation time is therefore not a critical issue.

4.7. Summary

Rule-based systems have a strong tradition in Artificial Intelligence research. They play an important part in human cognition as argued by, for instance, by Smith et al [51]. Especially for situation interpretation, rules bring benefits in safety and trust since they can be understood and verified by medical experts. Also they allow to tap into the vast amount of knowledge available from experts so that the costly acquisition of labeled training samples can be avoided.

	non-propriatery	supported by tools	expressive	shareable
nRQL	×	(✓)	✓	(✓)
OWL API	✓	✓	✓	×
SWRL	✓	✓	(✓)	✓
SQWRL	✓	(✓)	✓	✓

Table 4.4.: Classification of rule languages according to the proposed quality criteria.

The main idea behind the situation interpretation with formal knowledge is the concepts of Validness and Phase Specificness. A transition of a phase to another is considered valid if it does not contradict the surgery plan. The Phase Specificness refers to whether there is an activity in the current model which is indicative of the begin of a specific phase. Such activities are called Triggering Activities.

In this section four different rule languages to implement this idea were presented. To compare the options several criteria were defined. The solution should be **non-proprietary**, be well **supported by tools** and be **expressive enough** to elegantly represent the rules and make them **easy to share**. How well they fare is shown in Table 4.4.

nRQL is very expressive (and in fact contains a lot more abilities not relevant to this work), yet it is a proprietary solution, bound to a specific reasoner. Therefore, it is more difficult to share rules as they are restricted to a specific tool chain. OWL API suffers from the formulation inside the application logic of a Java program. This makes it very difficult to share. The knowledge is buried in source code, rather that presented openly and declaratively. SWRL has the issue of only being able to add assertions. It lacks the expressiveness to formulate queries. SQWRL is an extension to SWRL which precisely adds the ability to use queries, but not all reasoners support this feature yet.

In summary, no rule language fulfills all requirements completely. Yet SWRL and its extension SQWRL are very close. Both are actively developed and widely accepted standards and it is likely that they will reach a state of maturity where the availability of tools will no longer be an issue. Even now, they are practically workable solutions.

The evaluation showed that the approach yields to high recognition rate, runs in real-time and is stable. However, the impact of input noise has a strong effect on the recognition rate.

Another important part of the contribution is the formalization of laparoscopic adrenalectomies and pancreatic resections For context-aware systems, it is vital to have a profound knowledge, as emphasized in [8]. However knowledge acquisition can be difficult since numerous rules need to be formulated for non-trivial scenarios. Also, the surgery needs to be sufficiently standardized with few anomalies to expect.

5. Situation Interpretation with Experience-based Knowledge

In the previous chapter an approach purely based on formal knowledge was considered. Only knowledge extraction techniques were relied on to interpret situations. However, some knowledge is tacit. Not all knowledge can be easily articulated. This is especially true, if the surgical procedure is only loosely standardized or prone to exceptions. In these cases, people tend to rely more on their experience than on formal education as part of their cognitive process.

Therefore situation interpretation is performed with experience-based knowledge. As experience, annotated surgeries described with the representational formalism shown in chapter 3 are used. Methodically, this is realized with Random Forests. The concept is detailed in chapter 5.1, its implementation in chapter 5.2.

With experience-based knowledge also activities which are likely to occur next during a surgery are predicted. This can be used to issue warning before critical situation arise or to help surgical staff prepare instruments in time. This task is not suited for a rule-based treatment This is in contrast to phase recognition in standardized surgeries. There is usually only a small number of phases per surgery and the possible sequences in which they can occur are rather restricted. That is why they can be formalized in a surgery plan.

However, this does not scale to the level of activities. Activities are more fine-grained than phases. They are more numerous and can occur in a much greater variety of sequences. The individual activities of clipping, cutting and holding tissue can occur in arbitrary sequences and in arbitrary repetitions. The problem is more probabilistic in nature. For medical experts, it is very difficult to articulate and enumerate all possibilities.

That is why something like a surgery plan at the level of activities is not reasonable. For the prediction of activities in the OR the possible sequences are not modeled explicitly, but use experience-based knowledge and machine learning. Methodically, nGrams are used for this purpose. The concept is detailed in 5.1, its implementation in 5.4.

5.1. Concept for Experience-based Situation Interpretation

The core idea of the experience-based approach is to use actual surgical workflows formalized by the methods in chapter 3 as a representation of experience. This representation needs to be transformed to be usable as input for machine learning algorithms. It is commonly called a feature vector. Each feature vector is associated with a label. During its learning phase, a machine learning algorithm is presented with a set of feature vectors and their associated labels. This is called a training set. It is then to learn the implicit patterns and regularities between the feature vectors and the labels. Mathematically, it is to approximate the function which maps feature vectors to labels.

In the execution phase, the machine learning algorithm is presented new feature vectors which are not necessarily part of the training set. It is to derive a label which best fits the feature vector. This is done with a bias and the comparison of the new feature vector with the ones in the training set. Usually, some form of similarity is involved, as the assumption that similar feature vectors should be associated to the same label. This is a well-known approach for classification in machine learning and consistent with most of the work presented in chapter 2 and in [41].

For phase recognition, the feature vector $v = (a_1 \dots a_h)$ are defined as as a sequence of the last h consecutive activities $a_1 \dots a_h$ in a surgery. Alternatively, v is also referred to as the "history" as it represents the (local) past of the surgery. Consequently, h is called the "history size". The associated label of v is the phase the most recent activity, a_h belongs to. Thus, intraoperatively, when the last h activities are used as input for the machine learning algorithm, the (estimated) phase of the latest activity is obtained as the result. This is the currently recognized phase.

For the prediction of activities, the same feature vector is used, but with a different label. It is set to the chronological successor of a_h, i.e. the activity occurring right after a_h. Intraoperatively, when the algorithm is presented with a feature vector of the last h activities it thus returns its estimate of what activity will come next.

5.2. Realization with Random Forests

Random Forest have been introduced in [7]. Their fundamental idea is to use simple classifiers and boot-strapping to create a better overall classification. Specifically, Random Forests consist of a set of individual Decision Trees. The idea is to first train the trees independently from each other. Then, during classification, the results of all trees are aggregated and the final classification is determined by majority voting. To keep the trees independent each one is trained using a different, randomly chosen subset of the available training data and a subset of features. This also greatly helps with the feature selection problem as unnecessary features are automatically excluded.

The concept for experience-based phase recognition explained in 5.1 can be implemented with Random Forests. The idea is illustrated in Fig. 5.1.

The use of a history adds more context for the Random Forest to work with, in comparison to using just a single activity. This is important as the meaning and significance of an activity can change depending on the surrounding activities. This is likely to improve classification quality. Yet on the other hand, the dimensionality increases as more degrees of freedom are introduced. The size of the history therefore needs to be adapted to the problem at hand, but also the number of available training samples. The more of them, the larger the history can be chosen.

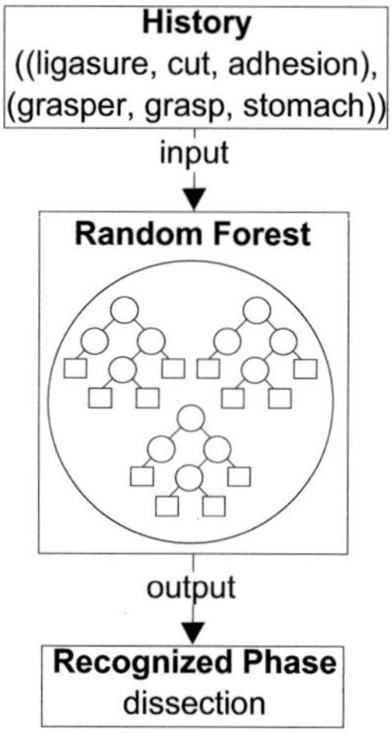

Figure 5.1.: RandomForest with a history of activities as input

5.3. Evaluation of the Random Forest-based Approach

The purpose of this evaluation is to quantify the ability of the Random Forest approach to recognize phases and the ability of the nGram approach to predict upcoming activities. The Random Forest is evaluated on the same data set as used for the formal knowledge and the same quality criteria were considered. This ensures comparability.

5.3.1. Evaluation Method

For the Random Forest approach, the same data set as used to evaluate the formal method is used (11 annotations of pancreas resections and 5 adrenalectomies). Also the same quality measures are applied (Recognition Rate, Confusion Matrix, variance and run-time). For more details see the explenations in chapter 4.6.1.

However, the evaluation procedure needs to be adapted to the fact that experience is used. It is impossible to use all annotated surgeries for the evaluation, since some are needed for the training. Doing otherwise introduces heavy bias. Therefore a leave-one-out cross validation was performed. All but one of the annotations are used for training, while the one left out is used as the evaluation sample. This is repeated until each sample was used as the evaluation sample ones. The eventual result is the average of the individual leave-one-out runs. This way a more unbiased classification is possible.

Since Random Forest are inherently random, the variance is of greater importance in comparison to the deterministic, formal approach. Each step of the leave-one-out cross-validation was repeated 10 times. This means that 10 evaluation runs have been completed for each evaluation sample. This data is then used to compute variance to see how the recognition quality fluctuates.

5.3.2. Results and Discussion

The recognition quality for pancreatic resections and adrenalectomies is shown in Fig. 5.3 for varying history sizes without distortion. As is evident, consistent recognition rates are achievable. With the pancreatic resection, the recognition quality increases with the history size h until $h = 5$. A similar effect can be observed in adrenalectomies, yet the recognition quality declines with $h > 3$. The reason for this is that an increase of h leads to more degrees of freedom which necessitates more training data. As only 5 training samples for the adrenalectomy were available and 11 were used for the pancreatic resection this result was to be expected.

With added distortion, the results shown in Fig.5.4 are obtained. They were recorded with a history size of 3. There is still a decline in recognition quality, yet it is far less pronounced. The Random Forests show to be far less suspicable to noise and outperform the rule-based approach even with little noise. However, it is also evident that Random Forests work better on the pancreas resection than on the adrenalectomy. This is not surprising since less than half as many training samples were available in the case of the adrenalectomy. In both cases the drop in quality is far less than with the rule-based approaches.

The confusion matrices are shown in Fig. 5.5 for the pancreas resection and in Fig. 5.6 for the adrenalectomy. No distortion was applied and a history size of 3 was used. As can be seen not all phases are recognized. The algorithm has obvious problems with port placement, closure and drain. The reason for this is that these phases are very short and contain only few activities. For the case of port placement, it is usually just one (namely (port, place, abdomen)). Since there are so few activities that belong to these phases, the algorithm cannot learn them reliably. The problem is accentuated with increasing history size. In trials with a history size of just 1, the system started to recognize these phase. In the case of port placement it learned the activity (port, place, abdomen) is indicative of port placement. However, the overall recognition rate dropped, since in the cases of resection and mobilization the context of a greater history size is important. Finding a compromise for the history size is difficult. The problem, however could be solved with additional annotated surgeries, as the Random Forest work well when given enough examples for training, as seen for the other phases.

The variance of recognition quality is lower for Random Forests than for the formal approach. They show a much more consistent recognition rate. It is in the range of 0.0003 for undistorted data to 0.0004 for a distortion of 50% for pancreas resections. This is two orders lower than the one for the formal approach.

The main reasons why Random Forest have a smaller drop in the Recognition Rate and a lower variance is that they are less dependent on individual activities, in comparison to the formal approach. Random Forest exploit information from all activities, while the rule-based ones only consider Triggering Activities. This helps to get more consistent results, since recognition quality is less dependent on the Triggering Activities staying intact. Also Random Forest do not consider all features with the same weight. More important ones are weighted stronger. Therefore, if only relatively unimportant part of the activity are distorted, the Random Forest is less affected.

In fact, Random Forests have the built in ability to quantify the importance of each feature. They are shown in 5.2 for the history size of 1. It is evident that for both surgery types, the most important factor is the anatomical structure being treated. This is not surprising, due to the nature of the surgeries. The steps the surgeon is performing are mostly related to the anatomical structures that need to be treated in specific sequences. The least important part of an activity is the instrument. Knowing what is being done to an anatomical structure is seemingly more important to the Random Forest than how (i.e. with which instrument). Therefore distortions of the instruments are likely to less affect the recognition.

Note that different surgeries will have different distributions of importance. This would be for instance the case when a specific structure is treated in several steps with different instruments. In this case, the importance of the instrument would increase relatively to the other factors.

For run-time, the system was able to perform recognitions in 0.5s on average on a custom laptop which is good enough for intraoperative use.

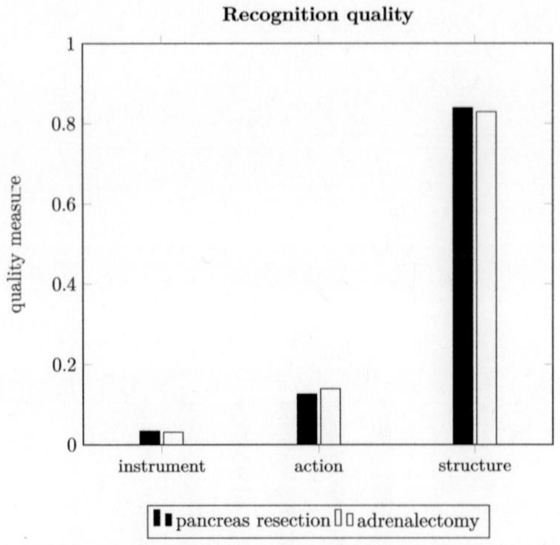

Figure 5.2.: Variable importance for h = 1

5.4. Realization with nGrams

nGrams originate from the field of computational linguistics. They allow the computation of the probability of a subsequent symbol to a given

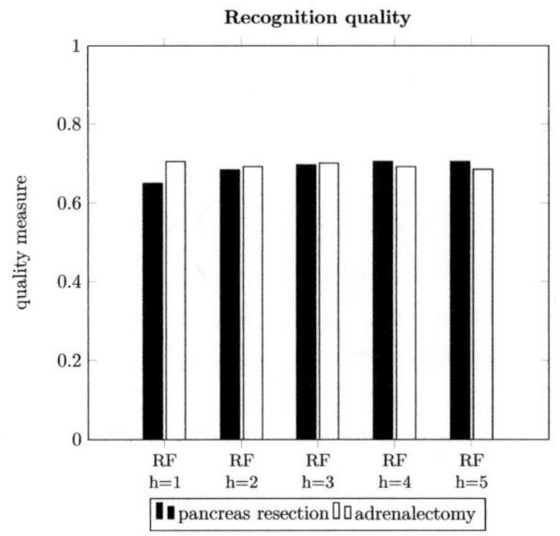

Figure 5.3.: Quality measure for Random Forests at varying history sizes with no distortion.

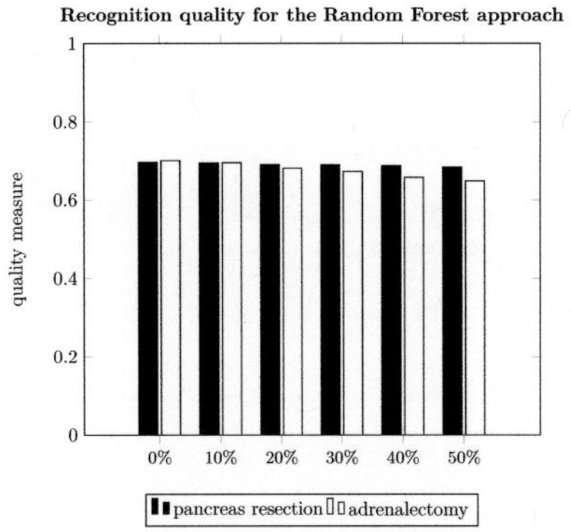

Figure 5.4.: Quality measure for all algorithms at varying distortion levels with a history size of 3

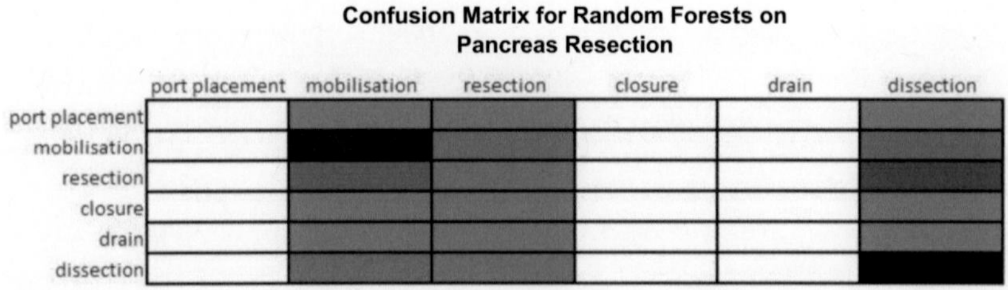

Figure 5.5.: Confusion Matrix showing which phases got confused. Darker values signify higher incidents.

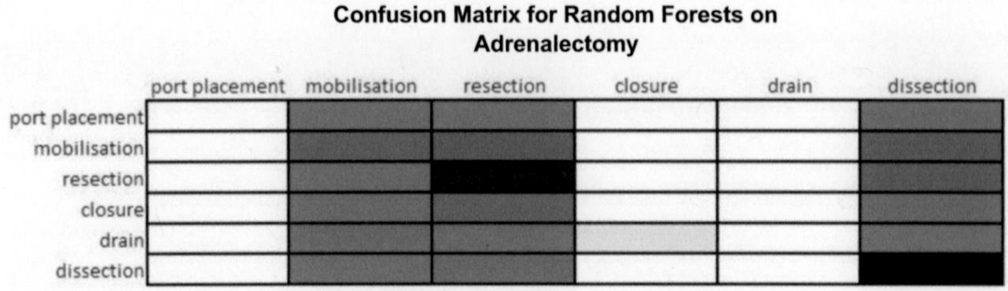

Figure 5.6.: Confusion Matrix showing which phases got confused. Darker values signify higher incidents.

sorted list of prior symbols. These probabilities are computed based on a training set of typical symbol sequences. In the field of linguistics such symbols are usually words, syllables or other linguistic concepts. In the considered case, activities themselves take this place.

The idea is that a history of the h last observed activities contains information about which activities are likely to occur next. Since there is a rather larger amount of possible follow-up events, it is not only interesting to find the most likely one, but to rank possible candidates according to their probability of occurrence. Fig.5.7 illustrates the idea. Given a history, several activities are predicted to gain insight in the immediate future of the surgical process.

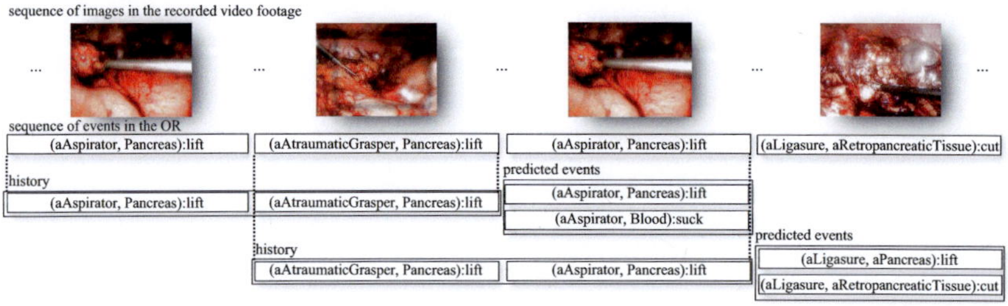

Figure 5.7.: Prediction of events based on previously observed ones.

Mathematically, the probability $P(x|hist)$ is estimated, where x is a follow-up activity and $hist$ the history of size h, i.e. a sequence of chronologically sorted activities preceding x events. For this purpose $c(hist)$ is computed, the number of overall occurrences of the history $hist$ in the training set and $c(hist, x)$, the number of times history $hist$ was followed by x. The probabilities for an event x given a history $hist$ are:

$$P(x|hist) = \frac{c(hist, x)}{c(hist)}$$

Prediction of follow-up activities is done by collecting h activities, matching the size of the history during the learning phase. Using $P(x|hist)$, the most probable candidates are identified. The values of $P(x|hist)$ are used as a confidence measure. This way, this system has a certain kind of self-evaluation. The higher the value of h is, the more contextual information can be exploited, yet also more training samples are required.

5.5. Evaluation of the nGrams Approach

Similar to the formal approach for situation recognition, annotated surgeries are used to evaluate the nGrams. They idea is to predict follow-up activities and compare them to the ground truth given by the annotations. It was published in [27]. The evaluation method and the results are shown in the following.

5.5.1. Evaluation Method

For the evaluation of the nGram approach, complete endoscopic footage of four different surgeries ($S_1 \ldots S_1$) were recorded. They were performed by three different surgeons. The considered surgeries were distal pancreatectomy and enucleations. The annotation was done by a neutral, experienced clinician who not involved in any of the surgeries to be annotated. On average there are 457 predictions per surgery, ranging from at least 171 predictions in S_4 and up to 815 predictions in S_1. To asses the quality of the proposed approach, the leave-one-out cross-validation was used.

The quality measure is the relative number of correct predictions and overall predictions made. That is:

$$\frac{\text{\# of correct prediction}}{\text{\# of overall predictions}}$$

At each occurence of a new activity, the system computes a new answer set, consisting of up to three most probable successors in this situation, as estimated by the system. A prediction is considered correct, if the actual, true successor activity is contained in the answer set. The prediction rate is then calculated as the ratio between correct predictions and the amount of answer sets computed (which equals the number of events in the annotated surgery).

sample	h=1, s=1	h=2, s=1	h=3, s=1	h=1, s=2	h=2, s=2	h=3, s=2	h=1, s=3	h=2,s= 3	h=3,s= 3
S_1	31%	50%	59%	47%	65%	68%	55 %	68%	68%
S_2	40%	66%	79%	61%	86%	91%	71%	91%	92%
S_3	32%	51%	60%	51%	62%	69%	59%	64%	69%
S_4	42%	66%	79%	60%	80%	88%	71%	84%	92%

Table 5.1.: Prediction rated with different history h and answer set sizes s

5.5.2. Results and Discussion

The results of the evaluation of the nGrams are shown in Table 5.1. Overall, a prediction rate of 80% was achieved using a history size and answer set size of three. For the most part, the system was able to correctly estimate follow-up events.

For surgery S_1 and surgery S_3 , there is a drop in prediction rate. This is due to the special occurrences in these samples. For instance, suturing only occurs in these surgeries. Such activities and their corresponding sequences are not found in the other training samples. This lack of coverage in the training data makes it difficult to successfully learn these patterns.

Reducing answer set sizes, decreases the prediction rate noticeably. This is to be expected. However, there is still a reasonably accurate prediction rate, signifying that the higher ranked events indeed have a higher probability.

The increase of the history size leads to better prediction results. Longer histories enable the system to make use of more information and a greater context. However, it also increases the degrees of freedom. This means that larger training sets are necessary.

Since most of the calculations can be precomputed preoperatively during the learning phase, there is little computational overhead when actually doing a prediction. This operation mainly consists of a fixed number of look ups in a hash table and can be done in constant time, far beneath one second on a regular PC.

A salient point which warrants further discussion is the fact that the evaluation was done under the assumption that a prediction is correct if the actual follow-up event is contained in the answer set. The answer set consists of up to three activities. The reasoning behind this definition is that it is very difficult to accurately predict the next event due to the inherent uncertainties of the underlying problem. Due to operating on the granularity level of activities, there is a high rate of variability in the temporal order and the number of repetitions of activities. For instance, at the beginning of the surgery, during the mobilization, the gastrocolic ligament is grasped and then cut. The cutting of the ligament usually cannot be performed in a single stroke. Several cutting operations are necessary. Oftentimes the surgeon also needs to re-adjust the position of anatomical structures before attempting the next cut. Therefore, depending on the surgery, cutting and grasping events can occur in arbitrary sequences, resulting in inherent insecurity about the next event. Given the available data, it is very difficult to guess whether another grasping activity will be necessary, whether the next cut can be done without a new grasp or whether the cutting of the ligament is entirely finished. Therefore it is reasonable system behavior to output several estimates of what might be the next follow-up event, ranked by their probabilities.

5.6. Summary

In this chapter, the use of experience-based knowledge for the recognition of phases and the prediction of activities was presented. Experience-based knowledge is useful, because one cannot rely on formal knowledge alone in all cases. Some knowledge is tacit and cannot be easily extracted. In this case, experience comes into play.

To represent experience, annotated surgeries were used. The vocabulary to describe the annotations comes from The Ontology for Laparascopy or LapOntoSPM. Methodically, Random Forest were used to learn from this experience to recognize phases and nGrams for the prediction of activities. The prediction of activities is important to, for instance, issue warnings ahead of time. This is an example of tacit knowledge which is very difficult to extract from surgeons. It is almost impossible for them to exhaustively list all possibilities. That is why experience is so important in this case.

To evaluate the phase recognition with the Random Forest a leave-one-out cross validation was performed on 11 annotations of pancreas resections and 5 adrenalectomies. The results were promising, yet not as good as the formal approach on undistorted data. The Confusion Matrices reviled severe problems with short phases. They only have few activities and thus Random Forests only get few examples for this phase. With a reduced history size, the short phases are recognized better, yet overall, the Recognition Rate tends to decrease. The long phases are recognized worse. A solution to this problem is the addition of more training samples for short phases.

When noise is added, the experience-based approach outperforms the formal approach. Random Forest are far less affected by noise. This substantiates the idea that experience works better with unexpected inputs.

However, the evaluation showed that the amount of training data is very important. While the robustness to noise is definitely higher with the experience-based approach, the Recognition Rate in the undistorted case is considerably lower, in comparison to the formal approach. Phases with too few activities are even more problematic. It also shows that the promise of experience-based approaches to be better in deviation and variations can only of fulfilled if appropriate training data is provided.

6. Combination of Formal and Experience-based Knowledge

Formal and experience based knowledge approaches have complementary traits. They both play a major role in human cognition. Unsurprisingly, there have been numerous attempts to combine them in so called hybrid systems in classic Artificial Intelligence [54–56]. Similarly, in the case of situation interpretation, one would expect a human assistant being tasked with managing assistance functions on behalf of a surgeon to be knowledgeable and well educated. In other words, one would expect him to posses formal knowledge. But with just formal knowledge and no experience, he would not be trusted in uncommon, special situations. A lot of human behavior is intuitive action guided by experiences. Lack thereof can have adverse effects. This reasoning is applied to the situation interpretation in this work.

The core idea behind this approach is to solve the problem of combination from two sides: the formal approach is augmented with experience and the experience-based approach with formal knowledge. The concept to do so is introduced in chapter 6.1, its implementation in chapter 6.2 and 6.4.

6.1. Concept for Situation Interpretation with Formal and Experience-based Knowledge

To augment the formal approach with experience, rules are extracted from experience-based knowledge. The rules can then be verified, extended and corrected by medical experts as necessary and expanded with the Validness Condition. They can be integrated into the formal knowledge. This serves to make the tacit knowledge contained in the experience explicit.

Methodically, the search for suitable rules is treated as an optimization problem. A quality measure is defined which quantifies how "good" a given set of rules is at recognizing the phases of a certain surgery. Starting from an initial set of candidates, a set of rules is determined which maximizes this quality measure. A swarm-based algorithm is used for this purpose, more specifically so called Cultural Algorithms.

To augment the experience-based approach with formal knowledge, the task of recognizing the situation is divided over a number of learning-based classifiers. The idea is that it is known, due to the surgery plan, which sequences are possible during the surgery. Therefore a specific classifier for each phase is used. It only knows about the possible follow-up phases. Thus the Validness condition is exploited to reduce the number of phases the classifier has to discriminate. For the purpose the idea of a Composition of Random Forest has been developed in this work. This approach has been published in [22].

6.2. Realization with Cultural Algorithms

Swarm optimization, sometimes also called Particle Swarm Optimization (PSO), is a computational optimization method [31]. It attempts to improve a set of candidates in regard to a given quality measure. This is done by "moving" candidates in the space of possible solutions. The movement of each candidate is not independent but influenced by "better" candidates, according to the quality measure and proximity. Additionally, they are guided towards the best currently known position in the candidate space, which is updated as better candidates emerge. This way, the candidates are likely to gravitate towards good solutions.

Such algorithms are mainly used in a continuous, or at least ordered candidate space, as this makes it easier to formulate the movement mathematically. However, as symbolic rules are concerned, a special variation of swarm optimization, namely Cultural algorithms is utilized. The basic idea behind this approach has been published by Kobti et al. [32]. It was originally developed to explain how cultures and cultural boundaries arise seemingly spontaneously. The idea is that people are influenced by their peers. The assumption is that the interaction probability depends on two factors: proximity and similarity. Physical proximity is necessary for there to be a chance of meeting. Furthermore, people are more likely to interact with people they like. These are usually people with whom they have something in common with, i.e. with whom they share similar traits.

Furthermore, the model assumes that the interaction leads to an increase in similarity. By interacting they adapt to the interaction partner in a way that increases shared traits. Practically, this is done by copying fashion styles, idioms or other preferences.

This model of development of cultures was discovered to be useful for solving optimization problems [40]. The population consists of representations of possible solutions to the problem. The similarity is defined as a measure of how well the optimization problem is solved. The idea is that individual candidate solutions interact with those who are already good at solving the problem and take on some of their features. Thereby, their chances of improving increase.

Candidates are defined as follows: each candidate contains a set of Triggering Activities for each phase. This way a candidate represent all Triggering Activities necessary to formulate the Phase Specific condition for all phases. If the Validness, too, is to be considered, it can be added to the resulting rule as described in chaper 4. Thus the tacit knowledge from experience is transformed to and combined with formal knowledge.

In the following, the initialization is described, i.e. the creation of the initial population of candidates is introduced. Afterwards the optimization process is explained.

6.2.1. Initialization

To limit the number of necessary iterations and facilitate good eventual results a decent initial population is essential. For this purpose, a heuristic is used to generate a sensible initialization.

The idea is to identify candidates for Triggering Activities based on some of their characteristics. Triggering Activities for a phase p will be concentrated at the beginning of p. Therefore it is computed how close activities are to the beginning of any occurrence of p in the temporal sense. This information is used to compute the likelihood $p(a, p, t)$ of encountering a specific activity a at a certain point of time t after the beginning of the phase p. This function is approximated by a sum of Gaussians. To determine if an activity should be a candidate or not the mode of each distribution is used i.e.

$$c = argmax_t p(a, p, t)$$

The smaller the value of c is, the more a is associated with the beginning of p. If it is under a predefined threshold, this activity is considered a potential Triggering Activity.

The initial candidates are created by randomly choosing Triggering Activities. These serve as the initialization for the algorithm.

6.2.2. Optimization

To perform the optimization, a quality measure must be defined. The average recognition rate is used for this purpose. It is the number of correct phase recognitions divided by the number of overall recognitions that have been performed. To evaluate a candidate, the Triggering Activities contained therein are converted into rules. Then the rules are applied to the annotated surgeries given as training samples. It is assumed that if a candidate performs well on the training samples, it will also work on new, yet unseen samples. As the termination criterion a fixed number of iterations is used. Alternatively, a threshold on the desired quality would also be possible.

The population is represented by candidates distributed over a two dimensional grid. The optimization is performed in cycles. In each cycle, it is determined which candidates are to interact to make the them more. The modified population is the starting point for the next cycle. For the initialization, the grid is populated with initial candidates.

In each cycle, the neighborhood of a candidate is considered. It is determined as the adjacent cells in the grid. The neighborhood represent physical proximity of candidates. The probability of interaction is 0 outside of it. Inside, it is proportional to the quality of the candidate to be interacted with, as given by the quality measure. In other words, candidates can only interact with other candidates in their neighborhood and they have a higher interaction probability with those who have a higher average recognition rate on the training set. The eventual interaction partner is chosen randomly, according to the given probabilities.

The adaption to the interaction partner work as follows: either an entire set of Triggering Activities is exchanged or just one of the activities. Both adaption types have the same chance of occurring. In the first case of an entire set being changed, the set for a randomly chosen phase of the interaction partner is used to replace the corresponding set of the candidate interacted with. In the second case, the set for a randomly chosen phase is altered with equal probability in one of the following ways. Either an activity which is present in the set of the interaction partner but not in the candidate is added, or one that is in the candidate but not in the interaction partner is removed. As the third option one activity is swapped with the other, essentially combining both former operation into one. The eventual result is the best candidate, aggregated over all iterations.

The approach offers a quick and efficient way to explore the space of possible rules heuristically. Checking each possible rule individually is not feasible. The number of permutations would be far to huge. None the less, this heuristic approach has its drawbacks. It cannot be guaranteed that the global optimum is found. The system might run into a local one. However, by design of the algorithm, the different parts of the grid can represent different "cultures". Cultures can be interpreted as sets of candidates which are similar and close to one (local) maximum. As numerous cultures can emerge, different local maxima are explored, increasing the chance that one of them will be the global one or at least close to it.

6.3. Evaluation of the Cultural Approach

As with the formal and experience-based approach annotated surgeries are used to perform the evaluation. To ensure comparability, the same data set as for the other approaches was used.

6.3.1. Evaluation Method

The same 11 annotations for pancreas resections and 5 for adrenalectomies as for the formal and the experience-based approach are used. Also the same quality measures are employed. Since, the approach entails a degree of learning, the leave-one-out cross validation was used to distribute the data over the training and the evaluation set. Again, 10 repetitions were done to calculate variance.

For the evaluation, the Triggering Activities were learned with the training data. They were augmented with the Validness condition and formulated as rules. These rules were then applied to recognize the phases on the training samples.

6.3.2. Results and Discussion

The recognition rate at varying distortion levels is shown in Fig.6.1. Evidently, it behaves similar to the formal approach. The results are good when no distortion is present, yet declines quickly when noise is added. The decline is somewhat steeper than with hand-crafted rules made from expert knowledge. This is also evidenced in the greater variance of about 0.3 for pancreas resection and 0.2 for adrenalectomies.

Learned rules evidently do not generalize as good as hand-crafted ones. The reason for this is that in the hand-crafted ones, higher-level concepts such as "cutting instrument" are used. In contrast, the learned rules only contain specific instruments, those which have been observed in training data. Therefore, the hand-crafted rules still have a chance to be correct if the distortion happens to change the instrument into another one that is sufficiently similar.

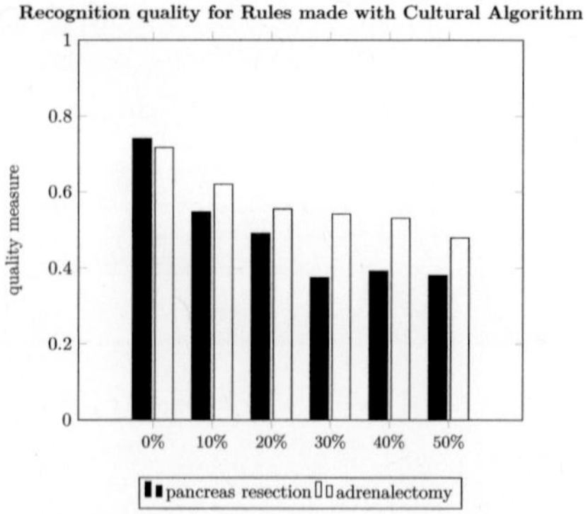

Figure 6.1.: Quality measure for the cultural algorithm at varying distortion levels

The confusion matrices are shown in Fig.6.2 for pancreas resections and in Fig.6.3 for adrenalectomies. As can be seen, all phases can be recognized. This is a major advantage over the experience-based approach which failed to recognize short phases. The reason for this is that the heuristic used to find the initial population explicitly looks for activities which are associated to the begin of a phase. Therefore, no matter how short the phase is or how few activities there are in the phase, as long as there is at least one, some activity will be found and included in the candidate set. The optimization process is then able to make use of the initial activity and use it to recognize all phases.

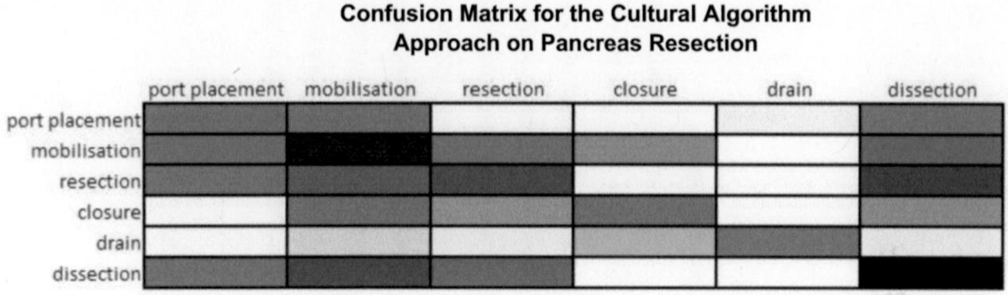

Figure 6.2.: Confusion Matrix showing which phases got confused. Darker values signify higher incidents.

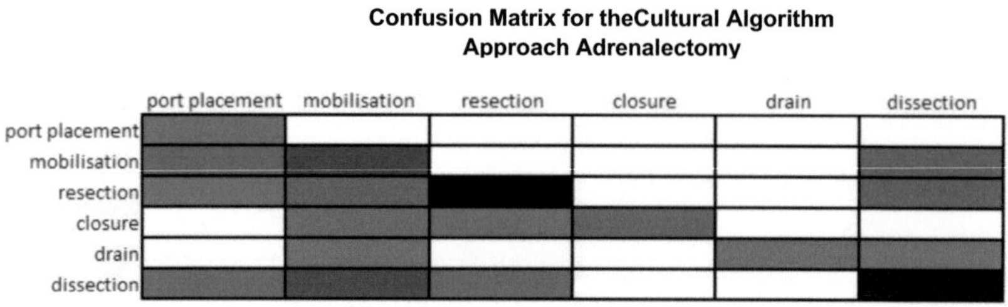

Figure 6.3.: Confusion Matrix showing which phases got confused. Darker values signify higher incidents.

It is also interesting to consider how well the optimization works. For this purpose, the Recognition Rates of the best rules found in each iteration are a useful measure. They are plotted, along with the Recognition Rate resulting from using all Triggering Activities from the initial set, in Fig.6.4. As can be seen the first step is the most important one, since there are already cultures which represent good solutions to the problem. Afterwards there are only little gains to make. For the pancreas resection, the slow improvements last longer, as there is more training data available.

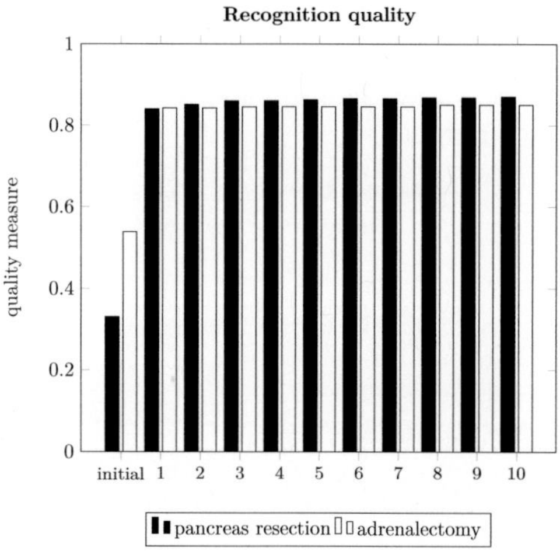

Figure 6.4.: Recognition quality at different iterations

Learned Triggering Activities of Adrenalectomies

Phase	Triggering Activities
Start	(Port, place, Abdomen)
Port placement	(Port, place, Abdomen)
Mobilisation	(Ligasure, cut, Adhesion), (Ligasure, mobilize, Liver)
Dissection	(Atraumatic grasper, lift, Greater Omentum), (Ligasure, cut, Dorsal Parietal Peritoneum), (Ligasure, blunt dissect, Gerotas Fascia), (Atraumatic Grasper, grasp, Gerotas Fascia)
Resection	(Ligasure, cut, Perirenal Fat Tissue)
Closure	(Specimen Bag, deposit, Resected Tissue), (Specimen Bag, grasp, Object)
Drain	(Drainage, place, Object)

Figure 6.5.: Learned Triggering Activities for Adrenalectomy.

Learned Triggering Activities of Pancreatic Resections

Phase	Triggering Activities
Start	(Port, place, Abdomen)
Port placement	(Port, place, Abdomen), (Swab, dab, Blood)
Mobilisation	(Ligasure, grasp, Splenic Artery), (Ligasure, cut, Gastrocolic Ligament), (Atraumatic Grasper, grasp, Greater Omentum), (Aspirator, place, Greater Omentum), (Ligasure, grasp, Stomach)
Dissection	(Ligasure, blunt dissect, Inferior Margin Pancreas), (Ligasure, cut, Dorsal Parietal Peritoneum), (Atraumatic grasper, grasp, Dorsal Parietal Peritoneum), (Aspirator, lift, Splenic Vein), (Atraumatic Grasper, lift, Splenic Artery)
Resection	(Ligasure, blunt-dissect, Retropancreatic Tissue), (Thread, lift, Object), (Ligasure, cut, Retropancreatic Tissue), (Atraumatic Grasper, grasp, Retropancreatic Tissue), (Ligasure, dissect, Splenic Artery), (Atraumatic Grasper, lift, Splenic Vein), (Ligasure, cut, Pancreas), Aspirator, lift, Spleen)
Closure	(Specimen Bag, deposit, Resected Tissue), (Specimen Bag, place, Cyst)
Drain	(Drainage, grasp, Object)

Figure 6.6.: Learned Triggering Activities for Pancreas Resection.

The rules learned when using all available experience as shown in Fig.6.5 and Fig.6.6. As evident, they are reasonable descriptions of the surgeries and could be further refined by experts. As the eventual recognition is done with the rules from the formal approach, this approach has the same run-time of 0.8s with SWRL rules.

6.4. Realization with a Composition of Random Forests

The use of Random Forests for situation interpretation has been presented in chapter 5.2. The idea was to have one Random Forest which learns to relate a history of activities to the phase of the most recent activity in the history. While this approach is certainly useful, there are some draw backs to it. The difficulty of the classification task grows directly with the number of phases. As there are more phases to discriminate, there is also more room for error. The underlying issue is that no information above the level of activities is used. In a certain sense, the Random Forest only considers Phase Specifness, but not Validness. In this section, the Random Forest approach is augmented with formal knowledge so that it considers Validness.

An issue that arises is that the result of the algorithm no longer only depends on the history, but also on the recognized phase. There is a chance that the algorithm will come to a "dead end". This could occur when a false recognition happens or when there is a deviation from the surgery plan. From then on, any future activities might make little sense to the Random Forest, as they are interpreted in the wrong context. Therefore, way of detecting and mitigating such dead ends is necessary.

The algorithm works as follows: For each phase p one Random Forest RF_p is created and the set of possible follow-up phases F_p is extracted from the ontology. For training, each activity in the training set which belongs to a phase $p_i \in F_p$ p_i is labeled with p_i. For all other activities the label $confusion$ is added. It signifies that an activity which is not expected in the phase has been observed. One explanation is that a transition occurred which contradicted the surgery plan. Another possibility for such an occurrence is that a false recognition was made and the system ended up in a wrong state.

To be able to get out of a false state, a monolithic, global Random Forest $RF_{monolithic}$ is constructed, whereby $RF_{monolithic}$ is a Random Forest as explained in 5.2.

During the recognition phase, RF_p, the Random Forest corresponding to current phase p (or in the case of the start-up the initial phase) is chosen and used to recognize the current situation. If one of the phases listed as follow-ups is recognized it is assumed to be the current phase. Otherwise, if "confusion" is recognized by the Random Forest, a mismatch is detected. In these cases, $RF_{monolithic}$ is used to reset the recognition. The structure of this algorithm is illustrated in Fig. 6.7.

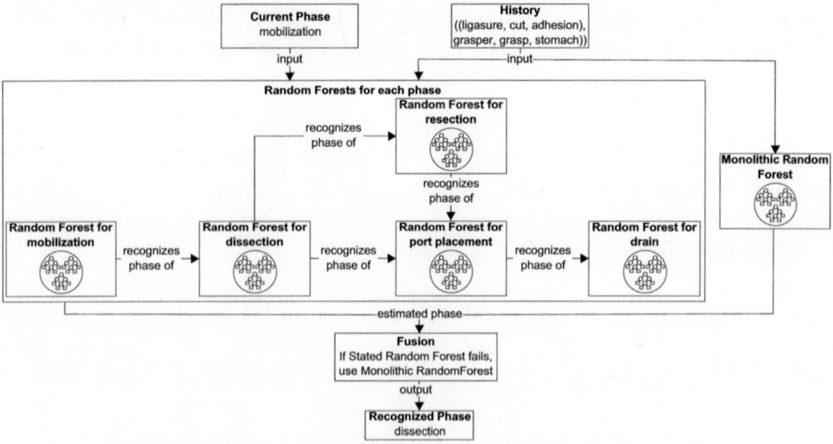

Figure 6.7.: Random Forest with Surgery Plan.

6.5. Evaluation of the Composition of Random Forests Approach

As with the previous approaches annotated surgeries are used for the evaluation. To ensure comparability, the same data was used.

6.5.1. Evaluation Method

As this approach is similar to the Random Forests with experienced-based knowledge, the same evaluation protocol was used (see chapter 5.3).

6.5.2. Results and Discussion

The recognition rates are shown in 6.8. The composition of Random Forests works very well in the case of pancreatic resections, yet fails to deliver satisfying result in adrenalectomies. This is due to two outliers. During the leave-one-out evaluation, recognition rate of 22% and even 0% have been calculated. With just 5 samples these two heavily impact the overall average. The bad performance is due to mistakes in the surgery plan combined with too few training samples to get out of a false state.

As for the comparison of the composition of Random Forests with the regular ones, the composite worked rather well for the pancreas resection. With a smaller history size, it achieved similar results and often even higher ones. For the adrenalectomy, it worked not as well, mainly due to the lack of training samples.

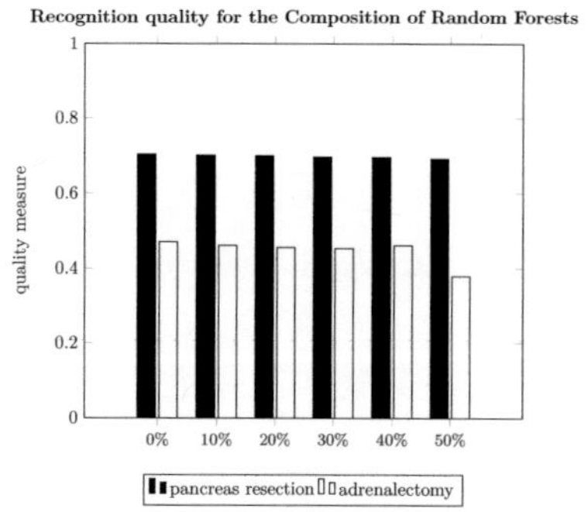

Figure 6.8.: Quality measure for all algorithms at varying distortion levels

It also suffers from the same problems as the regular Random Forests in terms of not being able to recognize certain phases properly. This is evident from the confusion matrices shown in Fig.6.9 and Fig.6.10. There is just not enough training data for the short phases to work with.

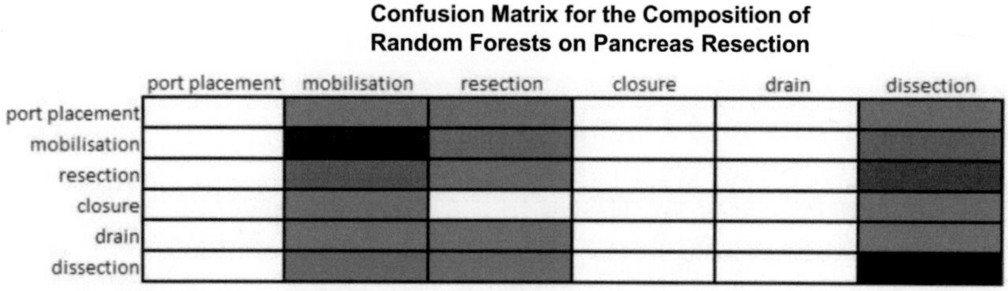

Figure 6.9.: Confusion Matrix showing which phases got confused. Darker values signify higher incidents.

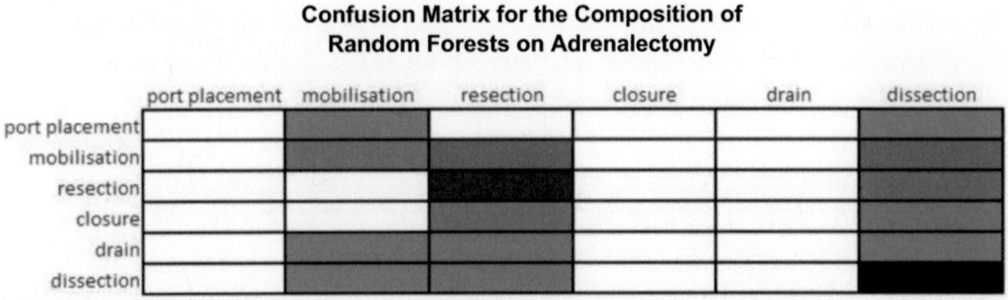

Figure 6.10.: Confusion Matrix showing which phases got confused. Darker values signify higher incidents.

6.6. Summary

In this chapter two ways to combine formal and experience-based knowledge were presented. All of the approaches to situation interpretation are summarized and discussed in the following.

The interesting aspect of the combination is the attempt of unification of the dichotomy of formal and experience based knowledge. Formal knowledge can be directly incorporated into the system. Fewer training samples are needed, in comparison to purely machine learning based approaches. This is of special importance in medicine as labeled training samples are hard to get. The labeling has to be done by clinical experts, whose time is valuable. On the other hand, medical expert knowledge is available from plentiful sources, from literature and clinicians alike. It makes sense to harvest as much as possible of it for the task of situation interpretation. Apart from these practical aspects, the formalization of surgical procedures has value in its own right. The medical science still lacks an universal, formal method of knowledge representation. Most surgical knowledge is represented informally. It is contained in literature or passed down from experienced surgeons to novice ones. Making the knowledge formal, explicit and shareable is useful beyond situation interpretation.

For interpretation with formal knowledge, rules are used. Rules are at the foundation of the oldest views on reasoning and there is modern-day evidence for the importance of rules in human cognition [51]. In particular rules lend themselves to application in the medical domain. They describe the relationship between activities and phases. Two different conditions are relevant when recognizing a phase given data at the level of activities. The first one is Validness: it states that the transitions from one phase to another need to be consistent with the surgery plan. The second one is Phase Specificness: it states that certain activities are indicative of the start of a new phase. These activities are called Triggering Activities. To formalize these rules, several rule languages (nRQL, OWL API, SWRL and SQWRL) were investigated. They were compared using several quality criteria. None of the candidates satisfied them all, yet SQWRL came very close. It only lacked sufficient tool support. This issue will likely resolve itself, as the field matures.

However, a purely formal based approach is likely to run into problems at some point. Some knowledge about phases is tacit, and cannot be readily articulated by experts. Moreover, deviation from the standard and special situation can occur during the surgery that have not been thought of when creating the rules. Here, experience-based knowledge comes into play. It is represented by annotated surgeries. These surgeries are used as input for machine learning, namely the Random Forest algorithm. Another medically relevant application of the situation interpretation is the prediction of activities which are likely to occur next. This problem was solved using nGrams.

To augment the formal knowledge based approach with experience, rules are learned from annotated surgeries. The method is based on cultural algorithms. The idea is to formulate the problem as one of optimization. The criteria to maximize is the recognition quality, as measured on a set of training data. The idea behind cultural algorithms is to use a number of candidates to keep track of multiple hypotheses. This allows the algorithm to better cope with local minima. Different "cultures" correspond to different hypothesis which are examined in parallel. Its main benefit in comparison to the purely experience-based Random Forest is that the learned hypotheses is expressed in human-readable form. The resulting rules can be understood, verified, augmented and corrected directly by medical experts. This makes the recognition more predictable and safe. In comparison to hand-crafted rules, it allows learning from experience and includes special cases that are likely to be forgotten by experts. Using it as a suggestion which is refined by experts is a promising way to deal with the problem of tacit knowledge.

To augment the experience with formal knowledge, a so-called Composition of Random Forests was developed. The (formal) knowledge about the possible transitions of phases given by the surgery plan is exploited to partition the task of phase recognition over multiple Random Forests so that each Random Forest only has to deal with a limited number of phases. This strongly simplifies the recognition problem. Since in reality surgeons can deviate from the surgery plan and the algorithm can generate false recognition, there is a possibility to run into a "dead end". To cope with such situations, a global Random Forest which does not consider the surgery plan, is used. It is there to reset the recognition if necessary. In comparison to the purely experience-based Random Forest, the recognition task is simplified. Yet the representation of the learned knowledge is still hardly interpretable by humans.

To better compare the approaches, the results are summarized in Fig.6.11 and Fig.6.12. Hand-crafted rules work best of all approaches in the undistorted case. However, their performance degrades quickly when noise is added. There is an especially steep decline from no noise at all to 10%. After that the decline is less steep, yet still very noticeable. The rules learned with the Cultural Algorithm work similarly. They excel in the undistorted case, yet have problems with noisy input.

Random Forest, on the other hand, are more robust. The Recognition Rate is hardly affected. The effect of the noise is more pronounced with the Adrenalectomy, as there are fewer training samples available. This is similar to the Composition of Random Forests. They are robust against noise and in the case of pancreas resections outperform regular Random Forests. However, they fail in the case of adrenalectomies. This is due to two surgeries which do not get recognized well. With just 5 samples, the variety in the data is not captured and the bad performance on these surgeries heavily impact the average of the Recognition Rate.

Apart from the average recognition quality, the variance is also considered in Table 6.1 and Table 6.2. For the pancreas resection, the Random Forest based approach are more reliable. They show a much more consistent recognition rate. The learned rules show the highest variance. This is not surprising since they use explicit terms instead of more general one. For instance they use concrete instruments instead of "cutting instruments" and similar concepts. That is why they highly depend on the concrete instance

algorithm	no distortion	10% distortion	20% distortion	30% distortion	40% distortion	50% distortion
handcrafted rules	0.0	0.037	0.023	0.03	0.026	0.0263
regular RF	0.0002	0.0003	0.0002	0.0003	0.0004	0.00037
Composite RF	0.0002	0.0002	0.0002	0.0002	0.0003	0.0003
learned rules	0.004	0.044	0.0366	0.036	0.032	0.0313

Table 6.1.: Variance of the quality measure for pancreas resection under influence of noise

algorithm	no distortion	10% distortion	20% distortion	30% distortion	40% distortion	50% distortion
handcrafted rules	0.0	0.0074	0.0062	0.00696	0.0054	0.0096
Monolithic RF	0.00035	0.00037	0.00061	0.0004	0.0006	0.0007
Composite RF	0.0061	0.0063	0.0137	0.006586937	0.015	0.018
learned rules	0.0021	0.0223	0.0237	0.026737315	0.0345	0.027

Table 6.2.: Variance of the quality measure for adrenalectomy under influence of noise

of distortion that occurred. The hand-crafted rules still have a chance to be correct if the distortions are sub-classes of the higher-level concepts. Also the Random Forest based approaches try to gain information from all activities, while the rule-based ones only consider Triggering Activities. This helps to get more consistent results, since recognition quality is less dependent on Triggering Activities staying intact.

Overall, the algorithms which rely on formal approaches, i.e. the purely formal approach and the learning of rules, work best in the undistorted case. However, they are suspicable to noise. In contrast, the more experience-dependent approaches, i.e. the approach with Random Forests and the Composition of Random Forests, are more robust towards noise. Yet they lead to worse recognition rates. This is due to their high need for training data. With insufficient data the general pattern of the surgery cannot be captured. Rare occurrences and variety amplifies this problem since rare occurrence are, by definition, only rarely encountered. A large body of training data is therefore necessary to learn them.

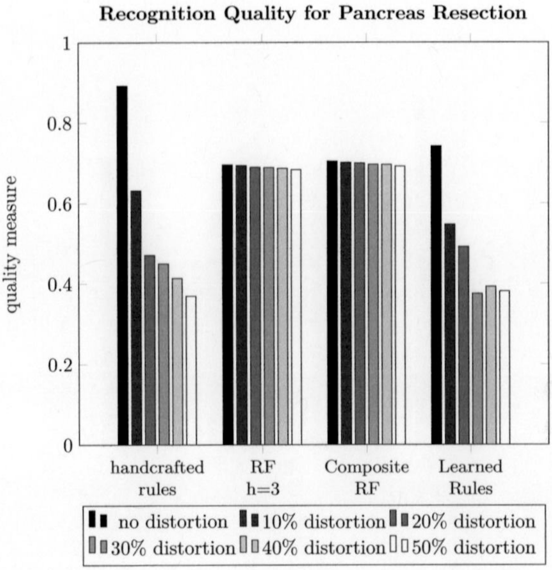

Figure 6.11.: Quality measure for all algorithms at varying distortion levels for pancreas resections

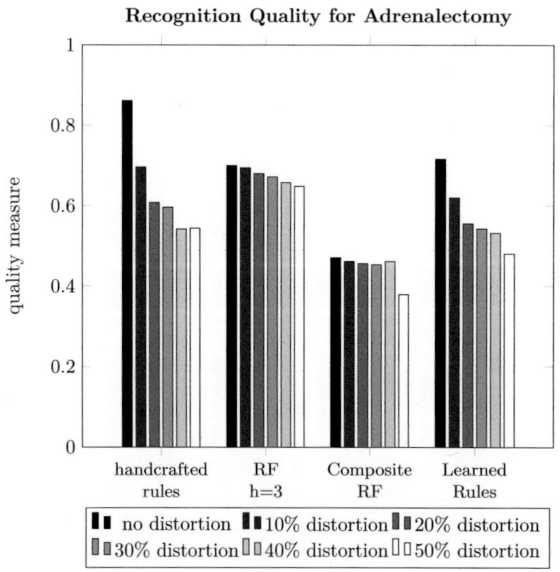

Figure 6.12.: Quality measure for all algorithms at varying distortion levels for Adrenalectomy

7. Towards Surgical Context Awareness in Laparascopy

In this chapter, the application of context-awareness to practical scenarios is illustrated. The surgeon receives Augmented Reality visualizations in real-time based on the current phase of the procedure. The visualizations are displayed in the monitor as this is the common way for the surgeons to perform the operation and can be implemented without bringing additional hardware to the OR.

For this purpose, the situation interpretation algorithms are coupled with MediAssist, a research system for image guided surgery. MediAssist does not provide activities. It only provides positions of the patient and the instruments using optical tracking. The challenge is therefore to recognize phases just from numerical distances.

This is done by transferring the numerical measurements to activities. This is closely related to the so called Semantic Gap. It is concerned with transferring informal information into a computational representation.

The idea of the approach is to map distances to the concepts "near", "medium" and "far". Is is then assumed that the instrument is performing an action on an anatomical structure if they are close to each other. This way, activities with instrument, action and anatomical structures are created from the data provided by MediAssist. Since the actual action is not known, the most general one is assumed: *surgical action*.

The algorithm to map the distance is based on fuzzy sets. They are learned from experience. This is a good example of tacit knowledge. For a surgeon it is very difficult to articulate what constitutes nearness or farness. But it can be explained via examples. That is why annotated example, i.e.

experience based learning is the better choice than formal knowledge. The general idea of the context-aware system was published in [18].

Using this technique two different context-aware systems for laparascopy are realized. One system aimed to assist during pancreatic resection. It provides warnings against risky situations by visualizing endangered vital structures, helps find target structures by giving cues on how to position the endoscope and assists by displaying the resection margin to support the removal of diseased structures. The evaluation is done on a silicon phantom liver to simplify the setup and allows to focus on the context-aware assistance. The experiment was performed with four medical experts. A structured interview was used to get their opinion on the usefulness of the visualization and of the context-awareness. This experiment is shown in chapter 7.2.

As an attempt to get even closer to clinical application, an assistance system for gallbladder removal on a porcine liver in a laparascopic training scenario was developed. Vital structures (the gallbladder and the gallbladder duct) are to be displayed when they are in danger of being harmed. The idea is to reduce warning fatigue by providing the warnings only when necessary, so surgeons take them seriously. This experiment is shown in 7.3.

7.1. Closing the Semantic Gap for Numerical Measurements

Numerical measurements are not only encountered in the context of Medi-Assist. Medical devices, tracking systems and similar information sources usually provide information in purely numerical form, without any ontological enrichment. One way of dealing with this issue is to include the measurements directly, as numbers in the situation model. This can be done using the Information Artifact Ontology, as described in chapter 3.5.1. However, numerical values are often hard to understand and difficult to interpret. A more intuitive way is to cluster values to linguistical concepts. For instance instead of declaring that a scalpel was measured to have a distance of 1mm to the gallbladder, it is often more convenient to represent the information as the scalpel being near the gallbladder. In this way, the relevant parts of the information are conveyed, yet in a more accessible and understandable way. By abstracting from unnecessary detail and clutter, a clearer picture of the current situation emerges. Therefore, methods to map numerical measurements to meaningful, semantic clusters and their inclusion in the ontological framework have been examined in this work. The concept and its evaluation were published in [26].

7.1.1. Concept for Conversion of Measurements to Predicates

At its core, the conversion of measurements to predicates is about quantization. A continuous set of real-valued numbers is to be mapped to a discrete set of linguistic concepts. The basic idea is to represent linguistic concepts as fuzzy sets. Membership functions which detail how strongly a given measurement can be ascribed to the specific linguistic concept are defined. In the instance of distance measurements, membership functions to linguistic concepts like "near", "medium" and "far" are considered. Intraoperatively, measurements can be assigned to the most fitting linguistic concepts and incorporated in the computational representation of the surgical situation.

The computation of the fuzzy sets can be done in several ways. In this work, three learning-based methods were developed to get the corresponding membership functions from annotated data samples: the evidence-based approach, the Bayesian approach with Gaussians and the Bayesian approach with Histograms. The training data consists of numerical values of the measurements and manually labeled linguistic concepts. The goal is to learn membership function which are then used to classify new measurements to the linguistic concepts. Furthermore, a clean ontological integration of these concepts was developed. The integration and the three methods are detailed in the following.

Evidence-based Approach

The evidence-based approach is motivated by the research of Weisbrod et al. [60]. The idea is to treat each training sample as evidence that this particular value belongs to the corresponding fuzzy set. That means information is used positively. New observations are used to enlarge the amount of real-valued measurements which belong to the fuzzy set. The membership functions for the fuzzy sets are represented as Gaussian mixtures, normalized to the interval $[0,1]$. For each training sample, a new Gaussian curve is added with a weight of 1 and a mean equal to the value of the measurement. After all training samples are processed, the function is normalized to the interval $[0,1]$. Thus, the evidence for areas with a high density of observations is high. Outliers contribute only little to their respective regions as they are too few to accumulate higher membership values. Given a training set T of real-valued measurements m, corresponding to the fuzzy set s, the membership value $\mu_s(x)$ for a measurement x is computed as:

$$\mu_s(x) = w \sum_{m \in T} e^{-\frac{1}{2}(\frac{x-m}{\sigma^2})}$$

where σ is the standard deviation and w the normalization factor

$$w^{-1} = \max_x \sum_{m \in T} e^{-\frac{1}{2}(\frac{x-m}{\sigma^2})}$$

An example is shown in Fig. 7.1. In this illustration, the sequential addition of samples to the linguistic concepts "near" is shown. With each addition more evidence becomes available and more values are added to the fuzzy set.

Bayesian approach with Gaussians or Histograms

Both the Gaussian and Histogram approach are based on the idea that $P(c|x)$, i.e. the probability of the predicate c applying in the current circumstances, given a measurement value x, can be used as a cue of how strongly the measurement x belongs to the fuzzy set corresponding to c. According to Bayes theorem, $P(c|x)$ is given by:

$$P(c|x) = \frac{P(x|c)P(c)}{P(x)}$$

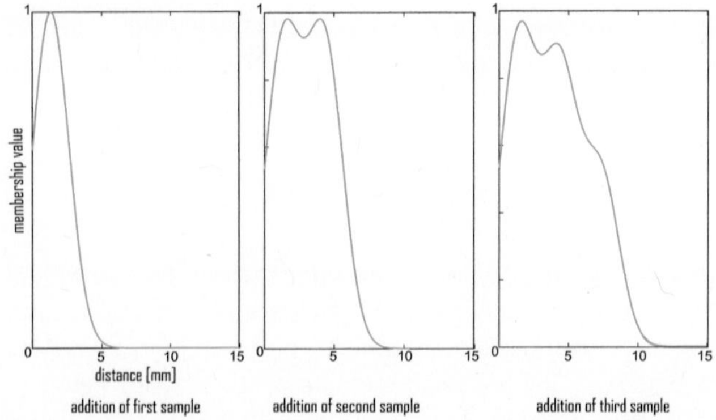

Figure 7.1.: Accumulation of evidence for the linguistic concept "near"

$P(x|c)$ and $P(x)$ are estimated from training samples. To do so the underlying distribution needs to be modeled. With the Gaussian-based method a normal distribution is assumed and corresponding parameters are estimated: the mean and the variance. The mean of the fuzzy set for concept c and the standard deviation ρ_c are calculated using the maximum likely hood estimation:

$$m_c = \frac{1}{n} \sum_{x \in C} x$$

$$\rho_c = \frac{1}{n} \sum_{x \in C} (x - m_c)^2$$

whereby C is the set containing the measurement labeled with c.

The histograms are presented with bins. The number line of the data is partitioned into equally sized intervals $[p_i, p_{i+1}]$. The number of distance measurements which fall into this range for each linguistic concept c is counted. After normalization, this yields an approximate probability distribution. It quantifies how likely it is that a measurement which falls into that particular bin is associated with c.

For the histogram-based approach histograms are used as an estimator of the actual distribution. In all cases, the resulting values are normalized to $[0, 1]$, to conform with the definition of fuzzy sets.

7.1.2. Integration in LapOntoSPM

To integrate this kind of distance qualifiers, first the concept of distance has to be integrated in LapOntoSPM. Being based on BFO, LapOntoSPM distances are to be modeled as relational qualities. They are qualities since their existence logically depends on other entities (the two between which the distance exists). It is relational since it depends on more than one entity. Since it is possible to determine the value of distance, it is a determinalbe and the concepts of "near" and "far" are determinated of distance. According to BFO, this is modeled using the is-a relation. In summary, the modeling as described in Fig. 7.2 is used to include these concepts in LapOntoSPM.

Intraoperatively, in order to incorporate the semantified measurement it is first assigned to the linguistic concepts. This is done using a correspondence function. Given the current distance between two objects, the fuzzy set with the greatest membership value is selected. The corresponding ontological concept is used to denote the relationship between those objects. Given a set P of linguistic concepts and equally named fuzzy sets the corresponding concept p for a measurement x is given by:

$$p = \text{argmax}_{s \in P} \mu_s(x)$$

This way the measurements can be cleanly integrated in the semantical situation descriptions. The resulting ABox is shown in Fig. 7.2. Other concepts besides distance can be modeled in the same way.

7.1.3. Evaluation

The idea of the evaluation is to quantify the ability of a system to recognize phases given the input of measurements, which are converted to linguistic concepts using the proposed algorithm,

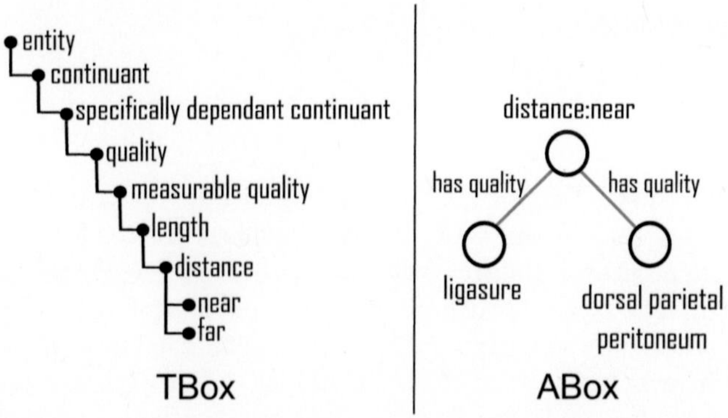

Figure 7.2.: Accumulation of evidence for the linguistic concept "near"

The general idea of the evaluation is as follows. In a phantom scenario with a silicon silver, the surgeon is to perform actions typical for liver surgery and the system is to recognize phase of the surgery. This way it is evaluated whether the conversion to predicates actually works for the intended task, the recognition of the phase.

The interpretation is done using ad-hoc rules with OWL API (see 4.3). The phases and their Triggering Activities are summarized in Table 7.3. The phase "treatment of diseased structures" is triggered when appropriate instruments such as scalpels are close to the relevant anatomical structures. Proximity of any sharp instrument to a vital structure, e.g. a blood vessel, leads to a "risky situation". All other situations are considered "safe situations". Due to the embedding in an ontological framework, all the possible cases are not represented explicitly. For the recognition of "risky situations", only *vital structure* and *tissue division instrument* are considered without naming the concrete ones.

Triggering Activities

Phase	Triggering Activities
Treatment of diseased Structures	(Tissue division instrument, surgical action, Pathological structure)
Risky Situation	(Tissue division instrument, surgical action, Vital structure)
safe situation	absence of other Triggering Activities

Figure 7.3.: Triggering Activities for liver surgery.

Evaluation Method

In this section, the method to evaluate the approach is described.

Quality Measure Using time stamps, the distance measurements in the evaluation set were played back, in real-time, and treated as actual sensor results. At a rate of about 1 kHz, the currently recognized phase was compared to the ground truth given by the evaluation set. The system's assumption about the current phase was constantly checked. The phase recognition was updated at 2 Hz on average. This quality measure inherently considers real-time requirements of the system. Cases when the system eventually recognizes the phase correctly, but takes too long to do so will affect the recognition rate in a sensible way.

Acquisition of Annotations The experimental setup is as follows: A liver phantom, an endoscope and laparoscopic instruments are tracked using the NDI Polaris system. Soft tissue deformations of the liver were not in the focus of the experiment. All registration processes were done rigidly.

Collection of training data Training data is needed to learn the correspondence between numerical measurements and ontological concepts. To collect it, a surgeon performed tasks as they occur in liver and gallbladder surgeries on the phantom liver. The positions of the surgical instrument were recorded using the NDI Polaris tracking system. The corresponding labels "near", "medium" and "far" were announced verbally by the surgeon. They were registered by an assistant by the click of a button in the recording software. All data samples were assumed to belong to the same label until a new one was selected. Of course, the on-line annotation leads to noisy data. The reason for this is the delay between the announcement of the new label and the adjustment by the assistant. Also, there are cases where the instrument only briefly leaves the intended distance range without the surgeon announcing it. Both effects lead to soft, smeared boundaries between labels. The collection of data can be performed very quickly. The recording of the annotated samples took less than 3 minutes, once the experimental setup is in place. Altogether, 1244 label-distance pairs were recorded. The process is shown in Fig. 7.4.

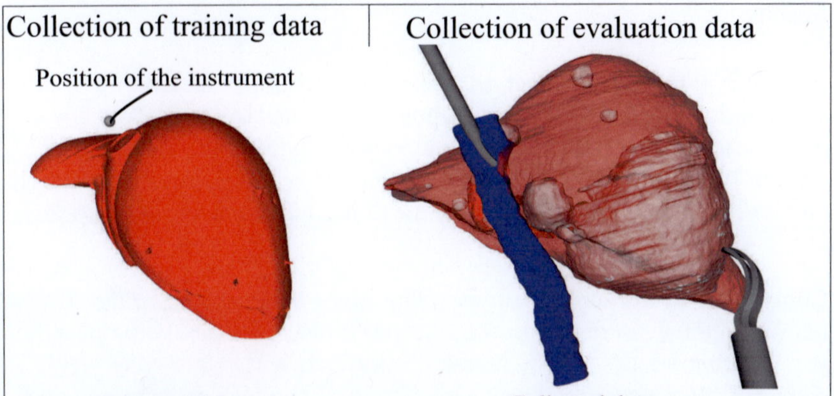

Collected data

type	value	class	timestamp
distance	1.33mm	near	9239ms
distance	1.14mm	near	9380ms
...	....	...	...

Collected data

type	value	timestamp	instrument	structure	phase
distance	216.42mm	5510ms	stapler	liverVessel	safe
distance	37.82 mm	5510ms	scissors	liverVessel	safe
...	...	...	...	...	...

Figure 7.4.: Collection of training and evaluation data

Collection of evaluation data Evaluation data is needed to asses the recognition capabilities of the proposed system. The evaluation set was obtained by having the same surgeon perform typical tasks found in laparascopic liver surgeries. This time, two optically tracked instruments were used. In further contrast to the training set, distances, surgical phases, instruments, anatomical structures and time stamps were recorded. The annotation was done manually by a medical expert with a own software tool, which was developed as part of this work, after the recording of the data. The eventual evaluation set contained 14,605 evaluation samples. The virtual phantom operated on was a liver with several tumors and vital structures as shown in Fig. 7.4.

The process to generate samples can be done in a matter of minutes (less than 3 min in the evaluation) and only takes negligible amounts of disc space (37 kB for the 1244 samples used in the presented evaluation). This is important, since customized profiles might be necessary for some surgeons to accommodate personal preference.

Results

In this case two qualitatively different results can be derived. For ones, the quality of the conversion of numerical values to symbols is a major quality factor. Secondly, the eventual phase recognition rate is essential. It combines the efforts of conversion and situation interpretation and is the medically relevant quality measure. Both are discussed in the following.

Conversion of numerical values The fuzzy sets used to bridge the semantic gap are shown in Fig. 7.5. As can be seen, all three offer plausible, yet differing results. The Bayesian approach with Gaussians yields to clear-cut membership values. This is due to the high restrictions on its shape. Since a Gaussian distribution is assumed, the only degrees of freedom left are the parameters for that Gaussians. Contrary to this, the Bayesian approach with Histograms makes only few assumptions about the shape of the function. On the one hand, this allows for a greater flexibility but also requires more data. Similarly, the evidence-based approach offers a high degree of flexibility, at the expense of required training data. In comparison to the Bayesian approach with Histograms, the resulting function is smoother. This is due to the underlying Gaussian curves. All of the considered approaches result in plausible descriptions of the linguistic concepts and are suitable for use.

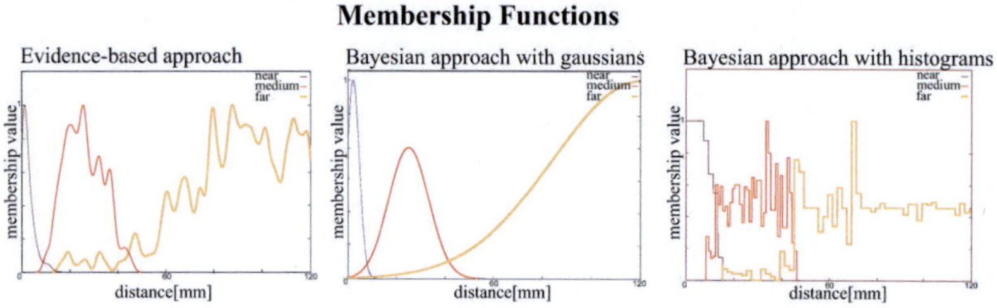

Figure 7.5.: Computed fuzzy sets for the conversion of numerical data to ontological concepts

Recognition rate For the evaluation, the samples were played back in real time. The distances were mapped to ontological concepts and the current phase was determined. The system's assertion was periodically compared to the ground truth. The recognition rate was computed as the ratio of the number of times in which the phase was recognized correctly and the total amount of checks made. Overall a recognition rate of over 93% using the evidence-based approach, 94% using the Bayesian approach with Gaussians and 97% with histograms was achieved.

7.1.4. Summary

In this section a way to generate and interpret a model of the situation at the level of activities from just numerical distance measurement between the relevant structures is presented. The idea was to convert numerical measurements into predicates like "near", "medium" and "far". With the assumption that an anatomical structure is being worked on when an appropriate instrument is near it, activities can be deduced from this information. Since the precise action that is occurring is unknown, the general *surgical action* is used. This way Triggering Activities and thus rules can be formulated to recognize phases.

For the evaluation training and evaluation data was collected using a silicon phantom of the liver. The ability of the system to recognize the phase was measured by comparing its recognition to the ground truth given by the ground truth.

Overall, the recognition rates were very satisfactory and appropriate for actual use. However, the situation interpretation was not perfect, neither was the classification of the numerical measurements. Most false recognition occurred at boundary cases, i.e. for distances right at the fence between two sets. This was especially pronounced for "near" and "medium". A large fraction of false discriminations was due to the those two. This problem can be solved by adding an additional set between "near" and "medium". This can help to better capture the space between them. Another source of false recognitions was the fact that the appropriate instrument sometimes was near a tumor just by chance, without the surgeon actually intending to do any work on the diseased structure. As forced by the rules, such situations were falsely interpreted as "treatments of diseased structures".

As can be seen in Fig.7.5 the membership values are sensible representation of their respective lingual concepts. The membership values can be seen as belief values. They signify the trust that can be afforded to the classification. High values for a measurement x translate to a high degree of confidence to the claim that x actually belongs to this particular fuzzy set. Low values, on the contrary, mean that there is no or little evidence to believe so. However, this is not equivalent to saying that x does not belong to the set. Truthfully, it means that there is not enough information to reach a clear conclusion. The ability to asses its own confidence level is a major benefit of the approach. It can, for instance, be used to refuse to map measurements to predicates if the belief values are too low. This could be the case, when the given value falls in a range which is not sufficiently represented in the training set.

Although some information loss is involved, the discretized computational model created by abstraction from the numerical values leads to a much clearer representation of the situation in the OR. It allows for the use of logical inference mechanism and discrete reasoning over real-valued data.

Note that the training data contained no annotation of the surgical phase. Only the concepts "near","medium" and "far" were annotated. Yet, still the full phase information could be interpreted. This is a great example of how the combination of learning and rule-based approach leads to elegant solutions. This way the number of training samples e kept low. Also the training samples are less complex. To learn which activities, i.e. which combinations of distance, instrument and treated anatomical structure need are indicative of a phase would require large amounts of highly expressive training samples. With the proposed approach, this is not necessary.

Another salient point is that values from the training set do not necessarily have a membership value of 1. This behavior of the algorithm is intended and desirable. It allows for noise in training samples. High membership values are accumulated only in areas with a high density of observations. Outliers in low-density regions have lower degrees of belief and are essentially ignored in the following processing steps. This is beneficial for the annotation process. If the annotator is unsure about a label, he can just take his best guess. The system will not place too much emphasis on this single observation by forcing its membership value to 1.

The differences between the three approaches also merits a discussion. The Bayesian approach with Histograms and the evidence-based approach have the distinct advantage of being able to approximate any distribution. However, they also require more training samples since they have more degrees of freedom. The Bayesian approach with Gaussians makes certain assumptions about the underlying distribution. Thereby, degrees of freedom are limited.

7.2. Laparoscopic Resection on a Liver Phantom

The purpose of this experiment is to use the rule-based situation recognition based on numerical distance measurements, as introduced in chapter 7.1 to create actual context-aware assistance and evaluate it in a phantom scenario. For this purpose the phases "safe situation", "risky situation", "treatment of a diseased structure" and "searching for a target structure" are considered. Specific visualizations were developed for each of them and are to be chose selectively only when needed. The experiment was published in [26].

For the evaluation, a silicon phantom liver was used. The experimental setup, the visualizations as well as the performance of the experiment and the results are shown in the following.

7.2.1. Experimental Setup

To represent the patient, a silicon liver phantom is used. An endoscope and the laparoscopic instruments are tracked using the NDI Polaris system. Soft tissue deformations of the liver were not in the focus of the experiment and thus all registration was done rigidly. With this the MediAssist system was able to provide numerical distances between the instruments and the liver. The setup is shown in Fig. 7.6.

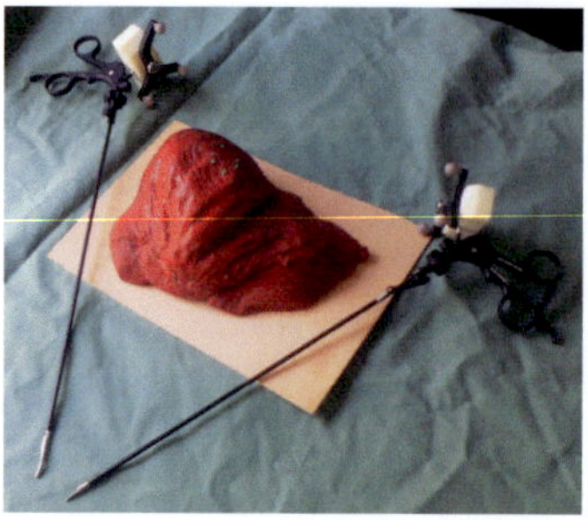

Figure 7.6.: Instruments and silicon liver phantom used in the experiment

7.2.2. Context-aware Visualizations

Three phases with need for assistance are considered: "safe situation", "search for target structures", "treatments of diseased structures" and "risky situations". The Triggering Activities for all but the "search for target structures" have already been introduced in Table 7.3. This new phase is assumed when the liver is not visible in the endoscopic image. This can be computed as the position of the target structure and the viewing frustum of the endoscopes are known. The corresponding Triggering Activity is then (endoscope, misses, target structure). The associated visualization helps get the target structure in view. All phases are then recognized using the ad-hoc rules with the OWL API (see chapter 4.3) and by closing the semantic gap with fuzzy set (see chapter 7.1.3).

The visualization for each phase are as follows: For "search for target structures" a green rectangle at the edge of the screen is displayed. It indicates the direction in which to move the endoscope to see the structure. For the "treatments of diseased structures", the resection margin of the tumor is displayed. Endangerment of vital structures, i.e. the "risky situations" is conveyed by displaying a virtual overlay of the structure. Its opaqueness increases proportionally to the proximity to the endangering instrument. Also, if the system assumes that the liver is about to be resected, it displays the preoperatively planed resection trajectory. All visualizations are shown in Fig. 7.7.

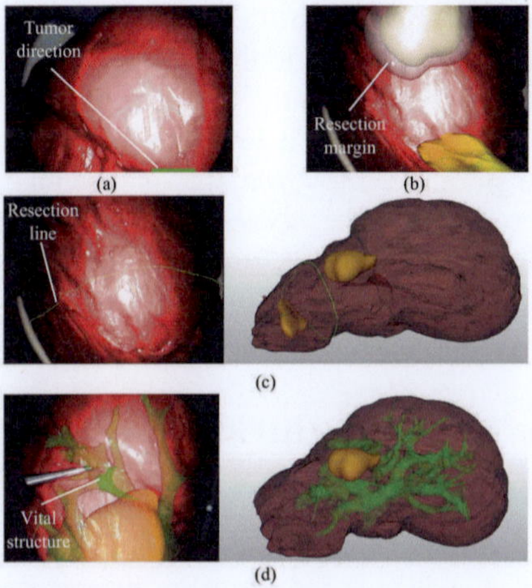

Figure 7.7.: Visualizations for liver surgery

7.2.3. Performance of the Experiment

The visualization was evaluated by presenting the system to four medical experts. In the presentation, the same experimental setup from the phantom evaluation in chapter 5.3 was used. After a brief demonstration, the experts were able to use the system on their own. During the execution, their reactions were recorded. Immediately afterwards, a structured interview was conducted. For the visualization, they were questioned about the usefullness and understandably of each. For context-awareness, they were asked if the visualization were displayed at the right time and whether they were distracted or inconvenienced by the visualizations in any way.

7.2.4. Results

The alignment of the endoscope toward the target structure was very well received. The visualization was described as clear and concise. It also did not take away focus from the clinician and it was pointed out that it did not disturb the view on the patient. The display of the resection margin was also judged favorably. It was suggested to add a visualization which emphasizes the overlap between vital structures and the resection margin. Particularly mentioned was the usefulness of the context-awareness. The vital structures being displayed only once they are actually endangered, was seen as a major benefit since it lowered the cognitive load placed on the surgeon. As a possible improvement, it was suggested to augment the cutting trajectory with the corresponding CT-slices. Overall, the visualizations along with the context-awareness were considered useful in the surgical setting.

7.3. Risk Avoidance during Cholecystectomya Porcine Liver

In this experiment, algorithms for situation interpretation are combined with a valuable visualization and used to perform a laparoscopic cholecystectomy on a porcine liver. The main goal of this experiment is to evaluate the medical benefits of the system under realistic conditions. In order to do so, a selected section of a cholecystectomy was performed on a porcine liver using context-aware visualization. The visualizations were aimed at issuing warnings about risk structures in the triangle of Calot such as the common hepatic duct and the common bile duct. The experimental setup is described in the following. The research was published in [30].

7.3.1. Experimental Setup

As the corpus, a box trainer by Karl Storz (Tuttlingen) was used. The original metallic underlayment was substituted with one of acrylic glass to avoid artifacts in CT scans. Furthermore, a common earth electrode was connected to the laparoscopic tower Fig. 7.8(a). As part of the preparation of the liver, the hepatoduodenal ligament was dissected proximally to the duodenum. Contrast medium diluted with water (1:1) was injected in the common bile tract. Then the common bile duct was ligated and the liver was positioned over the earth electrode Fig. 7.8(b). The caudal part of the liver containing the gallbladder was then exposed. To minimize soft tissue deformation, the organ was put under constant tension. This was achieved by suturing the fundus of the gallbladder to the soft part of the

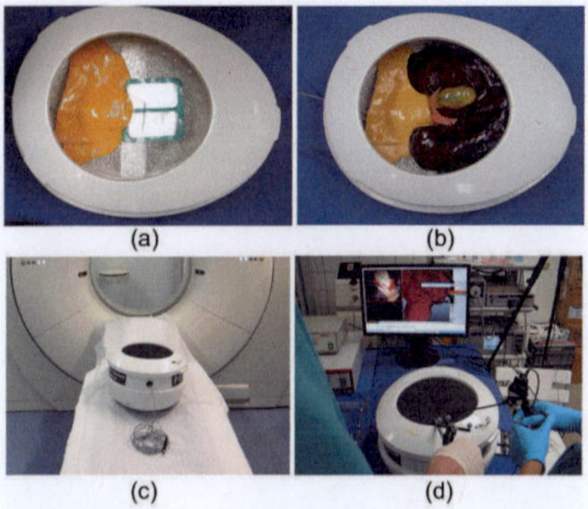

Figure 7.8.: Setup for the experiments: (a) common earth with underlayment (b) inserted liver (c) scanning with a CT (d) setup during the experiment

cover. Therefore, the organ was hardly mobile throughout the experiment. After the preparations, a CT scan was made of the liver in the box trainer Fig. 7.8(c). Afterwards the relevant organs (liver, gallbladder with cystic duct, common bile duct and common hepatic duct) were segmented using MITK [61]. A Polaris tracker was fixed on the box trainer and registered using rigid registration methods. The setup ensured a realistic setting and reflects established standards in laparascopic surgery. Intraoperatively, the instrument and the box trainer were tracked using the NDI Polaris system. The registration was done rigidly as soft tissue deformation was largely avoid using the described suturing technique.

7.3.2. Context-aware Visualizations

For this experiment two phases are considered: "endangerment of the gallbladder" and "endangerment of a vital structure". The vital structure in this case is the gallbladder duct. The phases are recognized using ad-hoc rules with OWL API (see chapter 4.3) and by closing the semantic gap with fuzzy set (see chapter 7.1.3).

The visualization shown to the surgeon are depicted in Fig.7.9. Displayed are an unaugmented view, as well as the highlighting of the gallbladder and the relevant risk structures, i.e. the gallbladder duct. Visualizations were chosen to be simple and intuitive, with a special effort to limit visual complexity while displaying them directly on the actual structures.

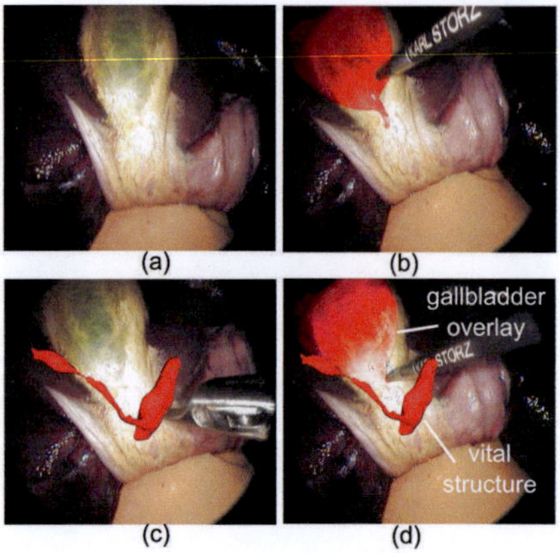

Figure 7.9.: (a) endoscopic view without augmentation (b) visualization of the gallbladder (c) visualization of risk structures (d) combined visualizations

7.3.3. Performance of the Experiment

After insertion of the endoscope into the box trainer, a pair of scissors initially approached the triangle of Calot to find the location of the risk structures. With respect to the visualization, the surgeon dissected the cystic duct. Scissors approaching the unclipped cystic duct lead to a warning visualization. Subsequently the scissors were exchanged with the clip. The clip was moved close to the common hepatic duct. This created a potential risk situation so that the common hepatic duct was visualized. Then the clip was exchanged for the scissors. They were brought closer to the clipped cystic duct which is not considered risky and therefore was not visualized. The performance of the procedure is shown in Fig. 5(d).

7.3.4. Results

To asses the medical value of the system, an interview with the surgeon was conducted right after the experiment. In this interview, the surgeon asserted that the system did help to dissect the triangle of calot quickly and safely without complications. The common hepatic duct and the common bile duct were not damaged. The context-aware visualization was seen as very useful tool to support the surgeon by detecting potentially life threatening situations during the intervention. Another benefit was the explicit knowledge representation which can be understood and the systems behavior can be anticipated. This also lead to increased trust in the system. Furthermore, the AR visualizations help with perception of depth, even in their simple form and with a steroescopic display. The simplicity itself was seen as a benefit to the usability of the system. Photo-realistic rendering additions such as realistic shadows or lighting effects were rejected, as the simple visualizations lead to less visual complexity. The accuracy of the virtual overlays were regarded as satisfactory. This is an encouraging result, as the registration only relied on CT-Data and rigid tracking without compensation for soft tissue movements. The visualizations were considered as intuitive, with their meaning and intent easily understandable. Overall, the interview, conducted after the experiment, confirmed that the considered section of the surgery can be performed faster and easier, compared to an execution without assistance. However, as an improvement, it was suggested to reduce the opaqueness of the visualization of risk structures. Otherwise visualizations may obstruct the view on important patient anatomy. This in some cases can even further complicate the surgery. Also there was a short, yet noticeable delay in the display of the endoscopic images. This was due to the processing time needed to perform the augmentation of the images. Surgeons, used to a faster display of images did find the delay troublesome. But overall, the delay was still considered acceptable.

In particular, these findings call into question the overlaying nature of Augmented Reality. While superimposing images on top of the actual anatomical structures is very intuitive, it can also be obtrusive. The general problem is that visualizations in the direct field of focus can easily disturb. Therefore, it is important to carefully choose visualizations and keep them as simple as possible. Also worthwhile is to consider alternatives where the visualization is not situated directly on the anatomical structure. This is an idea elaborated in the next chapter in the use-case of dental implant surgery.

7.4. Summary

In this chapter, the application of context-awareness to practical, laparascopic scenarios was presented. The visualization were realized using Augmented Reality displayed in the endoscopic monitor.

One problem in transferring the proposed approach to actual application is that the recognition of activities is still a matter of research. MediAssist, the image guided surgery system used in this work, is only able to provide distance measurements between instruments and anatomical structures. Therefore a way to map the numerical measurements to activities was developed. This is closely related to the so called Semantic Gap.

The general idea of the approach is to map distances to the concepts "near", "medium" and "far". An action of an instrument on an anatomical structure is assumed if they are close. This way, activities with instrument, action and anatomical structures are created from the data provided by MediAssist. Of course, since the actual action is not known, the most general one is used: *surgical action*. The algorithm to map the distance is based on fuzzy sets. They are learned from experience, as it is very difficult to extract such numerical boundaries and thresholds from clinicians.

Two experiments were realized: the pancreatic resections on a silicon liver phantom and the removal of the gallbladder on a porcine liver. The first experiment includes the evaluation of the attempt to close the semantic gap. The second experiment focused on context-aware warnings to avoid risky situations. The experiments are shown in chapter 7.2 and 7.3.

Using this technique two different context-aware systems for laparascopy were realized. One system assists during pancreatic resections. It provides warnings during risky situations by visualizing endangered structures, helps find target structures by giving cues on how to position the endoscope and assists by displaying resection margins to support the removal of diseased structures. It was evaluated in experiments with a silicon phantom liver. The experiment was performed with four medical experts. The structured interviews after the experiments reviled that the visualizations were, indeed, helpful. Moreover, the effects of the context-awareness were welcomed. The visualizations appeared when needed and were not considered distracting. Thus information overflow was successfully avoided.

After the experiment on the silicon liver, the assistance in a gallbladder removal on a porcine liver was realized. Vital structures (the gallbladder and the gallbladder duct) were displayed via Augmented Reality when in danger of being harmed. For this purpose, the porcine liver was placed into an surgical training device and operated on. Again, the context-awareness avoided information overflow and warning fatigue, as the visualizations only appeared when necessary.

Overall, the system proved its ability to provide context-aware assistance in a realistic laparascopic scenario. The evaluation showed the usefulness of context-awareness to avoid information overflow and warning fatigue. However, to actually prove whether context-awareness has a statistically significant impact on patient care large scale studies with greater case numbers are needed. This is outside of the scope of this work.

8. Towards Surgical Context Awareness in Dental Implantology

The work up to now has been concerned with laparascopic surgery. To show that the research is not limited to just one field, the methods were applied to dental implant surgery. Dental implant surgery stands to greatly benefit from context-aware Augmented Reality. However, fundamental issues of actual, real-world application, still need to be addressed properly. One major issue is the build-up of visual complexity by the introduction assistance visualizations. Most current Augmented Reality systems suffer from this. Therefore two major issues are addressed: superfluous visualization and occlusion of patient anatomy.

The issue with superfluous visualizations is that specific visualizations are typically only useful during certain phases of the intervention. The information need of the surgeon changes with the progress of the surgery. An example of this is the display of the dental nerve. During dental implant surgery the dental bur may get very close to this vital structure. Its injury can have severe consequences for the patient such as loss of sensation or pain. The display of the position of the nerve in relation to the drilling bur can therefore be very helpful. Yet it is only beneficial if there is an actual chance of harm to the vital structure. Otherwise, when the visualization is superfluous it can be irritating or even lead to warning fatigue. Similarly, the precise display of implant positions is highly useful when the position is actually being worked on. Showing all positions at once is likely to do more harm than good. The additional visual complexity adds too much clutter and requires too much focus. It is likely to distract from the actual work, i.e. the performance of the surgery.

The issue of occlusion of patient anatomy is as follows: the most straightforward choice for the position of an AR-visualization is to superimpose it on the object it refers to. In literature, this is known as contact-analog AR. For instance, it makes sense to display the desired position of a dental implant right on the spot where the implant is meant to be. This leads to the most intuitive presentation. However, by design, the virtual overlay on top of the currently relevant anatomical structure obscures the view on the important part of the patient. Such overlays reduce visibility on patient anatomy thus may even hinder visual understanding. An alternative display method is referred to as static AR. In this case, the visual display is in a fixed position in the field of the surgeon. While arguably not as intuitive as contact-analog AR, the view on relevant patient anatomy is kept free from virtual overlays.

In this work both issues are considered. Superfluous visualization is reduced by filtering using context-awareness. The formal approach to phase recognition with nRQL rules was used in this case (see chapter 4.2). Different versions of the visualization were investigated under the static and the contact-analog paradigm. The aim was to investigate the merits towards the the problem of occluded anatomy.

A a special requirement in contrast to laparascopy, is that dental surgeons are not used to see their patient through a monitor. Monitor-based Augmented Reality is therefore not apt. It adds additional hardware to the OR and heavily alters the established workflow of the surgery. This is why the visualization is provided via a see-through head mounted display. The calibration of such systems can be delicate so a novel calibration process had to be devised. It is introduced in chapter 8.1.

For the clinical evaluation, a porcine head was used to realize implant positions. All aspects of intraoperative application are addressed in this experiment: situation interpretation, calibration of the HMD and the actual visualizations. The system is based on [25]. With the experience gained from this version of the system and its evaluation, an enhanced, novel version was developed. All aspects were addressed and renewed. The research on dental implant surgery was published in [19, 23–25].

8.1. Calibration of Head Mounted Displays

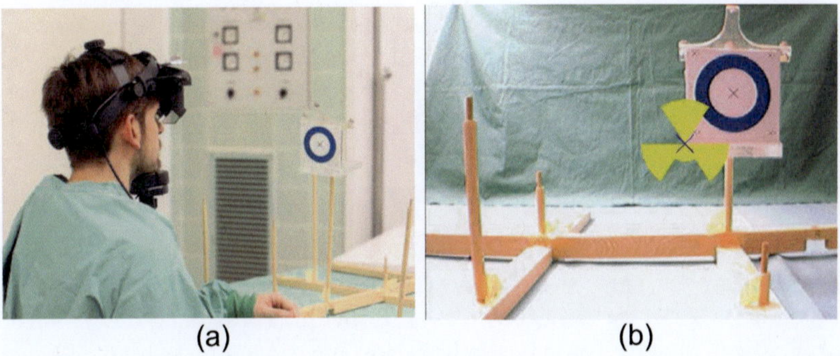

Figure 8.1.: Calibration of the Head Mounted Display from outside (a) and from the viewpoint of the user

The research presented in the following was published in [20]. In order to overlay virtual images correctly, details specific to the surgeon, such as the distance between eyes and other parameters, must be taken into account. Technically, the aim is to customize the virtual camera's parameters to a specific surgeon. The calibration method needs to be chosen with regard to the underlying HMD technology. The special issue in the case of the thesis is the use of see-through goggles. In see-through goggles images are overlayed on a semi-transparent surface in front of the eyes of the surgeon using small projectors and mirrors. This increases safety during system failure since the surgeon can still view the patient even if the systems stops working. However, calibration is rather difficult. In contrast to normal camera calibration, there is no footage of what the surgeon is currently seeing. Therefore specialized algorithms need to be employed in this case. A very common approach to calibration in such circumstances is SPAAM (Single Point Active Alignment Method) introduced in [59]. However, first experiments showed that the straight forward application of the algorithm does not lead to satisfactory results. Therefore a modified version of SPAAM was created as part of this work. It is introduced and evaluated in the following.

8.1.1. Modified SPAAM Calibration

The basic idea of SPAAM is to use real-world objects with known positions as a reference. During the calibration, virtual representations of these objects are displayed using the HMD. The positions are set relative to it. The HMD in turn is tracked by a Polaris optical tracking system. The surgeon is then to visually match both the virtual and real objects, causing proper superimposition (Fig. 8.1). The process is repeated until enough point pairs are collected. Regular rigid registration algorithms are then used to compute the desired parameters.

SPAAM was the algorithm of choice for preliminary experiments published in [25]. However, the results from the direct application of this approach were not as good as expected. To improve calibration quality, several criteria that heavily influence calibration have been identified. The calibration process was then redesigned accordingly. One important aspect of good calibrations proved to be the complete coverage of the work area, i.e. the area in which the actual intervention is to take place. To ensure and facilitate a proper coverage, a novel calibration object was developed, as shown in Fig. 8.1. Several different shapes and color combinations were considered to ease the visual superimposition and the most promising one was chosen (Fig.8.1 b). Another major source of calibration inaccuracies was the noise introduced from small head movements. Physiologically, the human neck is not very good at keeping the head completely still, especially for prolonged amounts of time. This problem is magnified by the somewhat heavy and cumbersome HMDs. To help reduce those unwanted movements a chin-rest was introduced (Fig. 8.1(a)). To further improve calibration quality, a subsequent calibration step was added. In this, the surgeon is to manually adjust a virtual chess board pattern to its real-world counterpart (Fig. 8.2). Thus, he can perform fine-grained corrections which can greatly improve overall quality. To guide the calibration process and provide an estimate of the expected results, a novel quality measure was developed. The fundamental idea is that changes in the calibration parameters should diminish as the number of point pairs increases. In other words, addition of new correspondence pairs should have a great effect on incomplete calibration and very little on already settled ones. Strong changes at the latter stages of the calibration process hint to poor calibrations. The quality measure also helps decide whether more point pairs are needed.

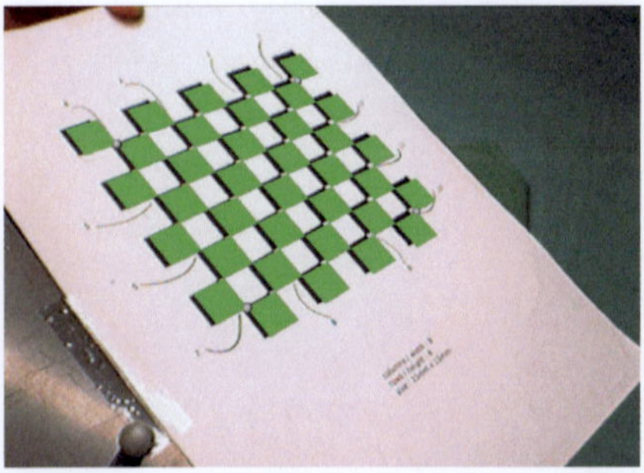

Figure 8.2.: Postcalibration process to interactively improve calibration quality

8.1.2. Evaluation

The evaluation of the calibration is a difficult task. In contrast to camera-based systems, with see-through glasses, there are no recorded images of what the surgeon sees. Therefore there is no recorded ground truth for the calibration. It is thus evaluated in practical application: the surgeon is to draw a pattern of points and lines projected via Augmented Reality on a piece of paper. Since the pattern is known, it can be compared to what was actually drawn. The error introduced by irregularities of the calibration is measured as the deviation from the original pattern to the actually drawn one. This method and its results are detailed in the following.

Evaluation Method

A user study with 15 participants was conducted to evaluate the quality of the new calibration approach. Each participant was tasked to copy a pattern of lines and points displayed via HMD on a sheet of paper as shown in 8.3. The drawings were later compared to the actual, true pattern. The experiment was done twice. Once with a naive SPAAM implementation and once with the new calibration process. The experiment takes all relevant factors and sources of error into account which would also be present in intraoperative use. It is thus allows realistic and sensible evaluation of the new method.

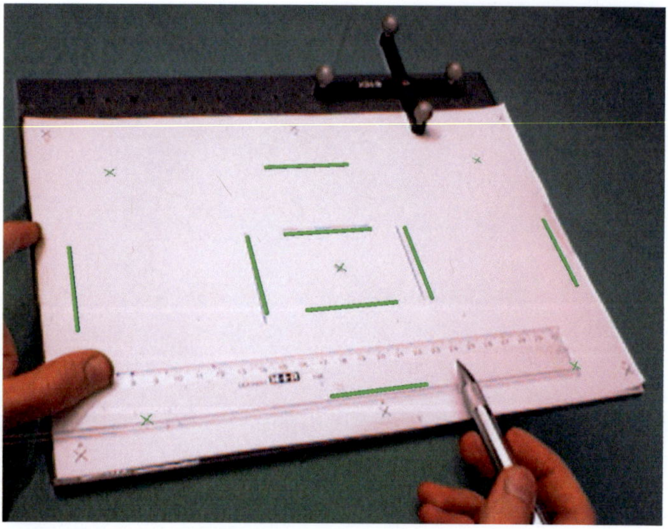

Figure 8.3.: Evaluation of the calibration by drawing a predefined pattern on a paper

Results

The evaluation showed that usability improved with the new calibration process. Most importantly, calibration quality increased for both novice and experienced users. Particularity the chin-rest had a great effect. Generally, it took less time and required less training or previous experience with AR to get usable calibrations. Average deviations from the lines and points in the pattern as drawn to the ground truth offer a quantitative insight in the quality of the calibration. The results are shown in Fig.8.4. With the old method, the mean deviation was 6.466 mm with a standard deviation of 3.46, whereas the new method had a mean of 3.01 mm with a standard deviation of 1.96. Evidently, the new method leads to better and more consistent results. To show statistical significance, a Paired Student's t test was performed. The p value for the null hypothesis, i.e. the equality of averages was calculated as 0.004243. Therefore, with a threshold of 0.005, the null hypothesis can be rejected. The improvements gained from the new calibration are indeed significant.

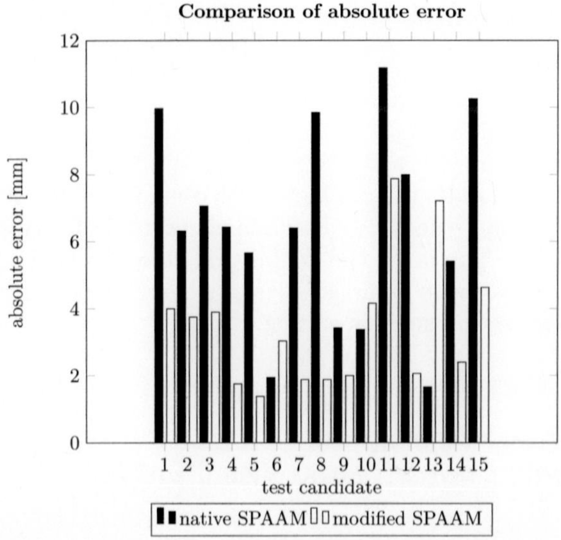

Figure 8.4.: Quality measure at varying distortion levels

8.2. Context-aware Dental Implant Surgery

The purpose of this experiment is to use the rule-based situation recognition based on numerical distance measurements to provide actual context-aware assistance in a phantom scenario for the use-case of dental implant surgery. For this purpose there is assistance for positioning the dental drill and reaching the planed depth. A warning is triggered if the dental nerve is endangered. The dental nerve is very important for the well-being of the patient. It is situated in the mandible and thus invisible to the naked eye. That is why it is very beneficial to visualize the dental nerve once the dental bur gets too close to it.

For the evaluation, a porcine skull was used. The experimental setup, the visualizations as well as the performance of the experiment and the results are shown in the following.

8.2.1. Experimental Setup

The setup of the system and the experiment is shown in Fig.8.5, with a porcine skull in place of the actual patient. The assistance is provided using a Head-Mounted Display, worn by the surgeon. Artificial landmarks are attached to it, so that it can be tracked using the NDI Polaris Tracking System. This way, the three-dimensional pose of the HMD is known intraoperatively. Similarly, the dental drill, the tray and the drill burs are tracked. This setup is medically plausible and could realistically be recreated in an actual surgical setting.

8.2.2. Contact Analog and Static Context-aware Visualizations

The system is meant to assist during dental implant surgery. The aim of this treatment is to provide dental prosthetic to patients with missing teeth. The basic idea to use osseointegration to tighten implants in the mandible. Osseointegration refers to the phenomenon that bone fuses tightly to some materials, e.g. titanium or special kinds of ceramics. For this, a screw made of the appropriate material is inserted into the mandible. Its position is carefully planed preoperatively. Using a drilling bur, the implant position is realized by drilling the hole in which the screw is placed. A special difficulty in the intervention is the presence of the nervus alveoaris, the so called dental nerve. It runs inside the lower mandible and can be harmed by the dental drill.

The phases were identified by consulting relevant literature, but primarily in discussion with clinical experts. The system is to assist in the drilling of the holes in the mandible according to a preoperative plan. The critical factors in this case are the position, depth and alignment of the dental drill in relation to the intended implants. The second phase is about avoidance of injury of the nervus alveolaris. The system should display a visual warning if the drill is likely to harm the nerve. Finally, the system should assist during the change of the drill head. The idea is to show the surgeon the currently used drilling bur and the ones to be used in the future.

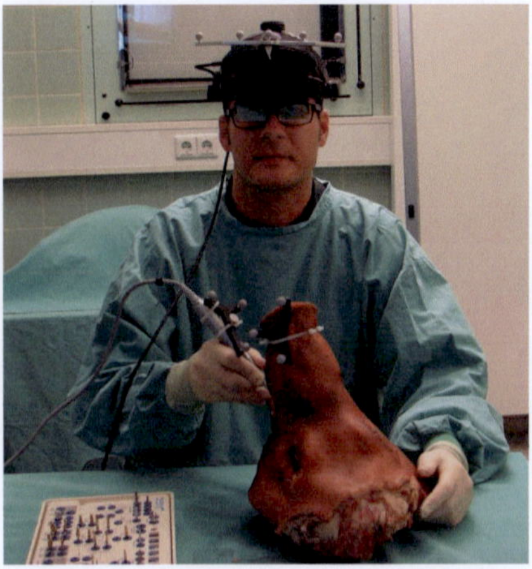

Figure 8.5.: Experimental setup for the experiment

Visualizations were chosen and designed with patient outcome and safety in mind. For every required piece of information, there is one visualization using contact analog AR and another with static AR. The idea is to give surgeons the choice between the more intuitive contact analog version and the less intrusive static AR. Therefore, each surgeon can make his own trade-off for each visualization. Figure 8.6(a) shows current alignment and depth of the dental drill in relation to the planning data. The deviation is color-coded. Red and yellow denote large deviations (Fig. 8.6(a)), green signifies small ones (Fig. 8.6(b)). Figure 8.6(c) shows the warning issued when the nervus alveolaris is threatened. In the contact analog version, the nerve and the tip of the drill as well as their distance, is visualized in the left corner of the surgeon's view, in the AR version the same information is overlaid over the real structures. Lastly, the instrument tray along with the used and upcoming drill heads is visualized (Fig. 8.6(d)).

8.2.3. Performance of the Experiment

The get insight into how the system performs in actual application, an experiment was conducted where a surgeon placed implant positions in the mandible of a porcine skull. First, Cone-Beam CT images of the porcine

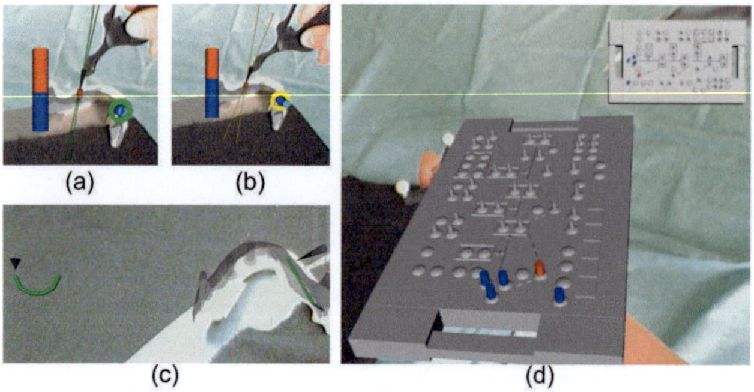

Figure 8.6.: Contact analog and static visualization for dental implant surgery

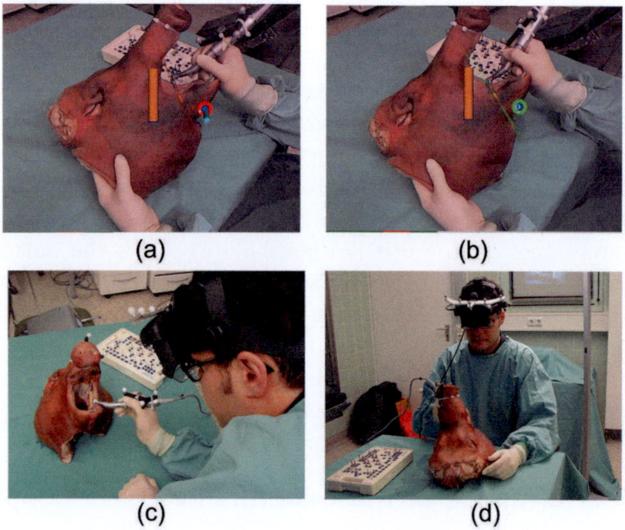

Figure 8.7.: Performance of the experiment

were taken and segmented. The segmentation was done semi-automatically, as only bone structures needed to be identified. A rendering is shown in Fig.8.8. The results were used to plan two implant positions in the mandible. The experimental setup is shown in Fig. 8.7 (c) and (d): the surgeon is equipped with a HMD, tracked by the NDI Polaris system. Positions of the dental drill, drill heads and implants were tracked in the same way. The surgeon's task was to place two implants in the mandible. The process was assistanted with context-aware AR visualizations, as shown in 8.7 (a) and (b). After the intervention, the surgeon answered a questionnaire which was aimed to judge medical merits and applicability.

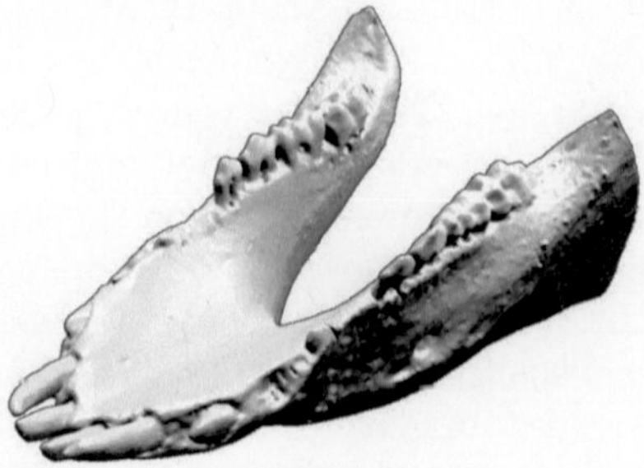

Figure 8.8.: Segmented scan of the porcine mandible

8.2.4. Results

In the following, the results of this evaluation are presented. First, the quality of the calibration and the accuracy of the realized implant positions are considered. Afterwards, the usability and medical merits of the system are discussed. This is the major point of the evaluation. The aspect of context-awareness takes precedence over mechanical accuracy.

Accuracy of implant placement To compare the placed implant positions against the planing, a postoperative cone-beam-CT was taken and registered to the preoperative data set. The first implant position was realized with a deviation of 1.1 mm and 2 degrees. Thus, the results for this implant position were satisfactory. During the drilling at the second position, the surgeon encountered problems due to a deciduous tooth beneath the intended position. This went unrecognized during the planning process. Therefore, this position could not be realized correctly. There was a positional deviation of 2.48 mm. The alignment could not be assessed since no clear hole could form.

Usability The questionnaire showed the usefulness of context-awareness AR in this intervention. Particularly, the participating surgeon agreed to the statement that the system overall made the performance of the surgery easier and less stressful. Especially the display of the drill axis in relation to the intended implant was regraded as beneficial, and so was the color coding of the deviation. The static version with the top-down view allowed the surgeon to align the dental drill without moving his head. This made it easier to get a different perspective on the scene. It changed and simplified the intraoperative workflow and showed ergonomical advantage. Nonetheless, the additional display of the axis for visual verification was still appreciated. The visualization of the nervus alveolaris helped to avoid injury. The nerve remained undamaged during the experiments. However, the surgeon purposefully restricted himself to a greater safety margin than the one visualized by the system to be on the safe side. The display of device specific data, such as engine torque and speed was missed. Apart from that, all currently relevant information was available and displayed in a clear and intuitive way. Generally, the static version was preferred in comparison to contact analog AR. The surgeon preferred its clear view on the patient in combination with a simpler representation of information.

8.3. Summary

In this chapter, the application of the knowledge based approach to phase recognition in dental implant surgery was shown. The visualizations were realized using a see-through head mounted display. For this type of visualization modality, the calibration is very difficult. Therefore a modified SPAAM-based approach was developed to calibrate the device in a medical setting.

With this, implant positions were realized on a porcine skull. Special emphasis was put on reducing superfluous visualizations and occlusion of patient anatomy. Superfluous visualizations where avoided by recognizing the phase and displaying only what is relevant in that particular phase. The formal knowledge approach with nRQL was used for that purpose (see chapter 4.2). Occlusion of patient anatomy was handled by providing an alternative to contact-analog visualizations, which are displayed on top of patient anatomy. The alternative is static Augmented Reality displayed in a fixed region in the view of the surgeon.

The experiment on the porcine skull proves the feasibility of the proposed system for navigation and avoidance of risky situations. The system leads to improved working conditions, as reported by the participating surgeon. Information is provided intuitively, right in the surgeon's field of view. The surgeon can keep his eyes on the patient for the entire surgery, without having to look away to see monitors. This is very likely to decrease intervention time and improve safety. Yet further work is necessary to prove and quantify the effect. The system also helped with spacial awareness. For instance, the nervus alveolaris, sitting underneath bone structures, was made visible. Combined with the automatic adaption to the current context, the proposed approach allows the surgeon to make full use of all available information with minimal effort. During the experiments, the system enjoyed great acceptance. It was perceived as a helpful assistant, rather than a device which requires training and concentration. Another benefit of the systems is the increased flexibility. The preoperative planning is readily available, yet the surgeon is free to deviate from it. However, it must be said that the results are somewhat weakened by the fact that these assertions were only attained from one participating surgeon.

The occlusion of patient anatomy by virtual overlays is countered with the alternative static visualization. The problem of sensory overload is handled with context-awareness. Even with the simple distance measurement, all phases were correctly captured. Furthermore, the phases were sufficiently separable for the proposed rule-based approach to work.

Accuracy, on the other hand, was not satisfactory. The measured deviation of up to 3 mm is not enough for clinical use. The NDI Polaris system does allow for very precise measurements, yet the calibration and the combination of several different measurements leads to an accumulation of errors. While there are possible approaches like the fusion of the Polaris measurements with accelerometers, this is not the purpose of this work. The experiments showed the applicability and usefulness of context-aware Augmented Reality for dental implant surgery.

9. Conclusion

The goal of this work was to develop methods for knowledge-based recognition of surgical phases and use it to provide intraoperative context-aware Augmented Reality. For this purposes, the use of formal and experience-based knowledge was investigated. Formal knowledge is the type of knowledge found in literature and university lectures, experience-based knowledge corresponds to observation of actual real world events. Methods using each knowledge type exclusively and methods using a combination thereof to recognize surgical phases have been considered. Clinical applicability was shown in the context-aware removal of the gallbladder of a porcine liver and the realization of dental implant positions in a porcine skull. In both cases, Augmented Reality visualization have been developed as part of this thesis. In the following the contributions and results of the work are summarized and discussed.

9.1. Summary and Discussion

In this work, several contributions in regards of formal and experience-based knowledge representation, interpretation and context-aware assistance with Augmented Reality were made. The contributions in each aspect are summarized and discussed in the following.

Representation of formal knowledge The idea behind formal knowledge representation is to represent all formal knowledge, e.g. from books, lectures and medical experts, in a generic, computational way. It is used in two ways: to support situation interpretation by making the interpreter more knowledgeable and to represent experience-based knowledge.

To represent the knowledge several requirements were derived: adequate completeness, reusability and real-time capability. Since reusability and real-time capability are conflicting requirements, two ontologies were developed: The Ontology for Laparascopy and LapOntoSPM.

The Ontology for Laprascopy is a custom-tailored solution for intraoperative situation interpretation. It is adequately complete and fast, yet difficult to reuse. No upper-ontology was used and no other ontologies are integrated. That is why this ontology is not embedded in larger frameworks and thus difficult to reuse. LapOntoSPM, on the other hand, uses the well-established upper-ontology BFO and incorporates several standard ontologies (The Foundation Model of Anatomy, the Information Artifact Ontology and the Unit Ontology). Apart from being reusable, it contains more semantic content. However, reasoning services take longer.

The knowledge representation allows to recognize all phases in the considered surgery types. Especially with LapOntoSPM, the knowledge is represented in a standardized way and easy to reuse and share.

Representation of experience-based knowledge Being knowledgeable is not enough. In most practical scenarios, experience plays a major role. To represent experience-based knowledge, formal descriptions of observed workflows were used. The idea is to record endoscopic video footage from real surgeries and annotate the activities and phases. This information about the surgical workflow is then translated into a formal representation using the vocabulary and representational formalism given by the formal knowledge representation.

Both knowledge types are linked. This means that for instance, if a specific scalpel is used in a surgery, all its functional properties such as its ability to cut can be automatically inferred from the general knowledge about the abstract concept "scalpel".

For this purpose two different approaches for The Ontology for Laparascopy were developed and contrasted: the isolated and the connected one. The isolated approach is only concerned with the representation of a single situation, i.e. the set of activities currently occurring in the OR. The connected approach connects the current situation and represents the entire workflow over time. Since the major point of The Ontology For

Laparascopy is the real-time requirement, the isolated approach was used as it makes the representation simpler.

LapOntoSPM adheres to established standards. The modeling is compatible with the upper-ontology BFO and the core ontology OntoSPM. This allows for easier sharing of knowledge and reusabilty. However, due to the richer representation run-time for reasoning is affected.

Knowledge-based Situation Interpretation The idea behind knowledge-based situation interpretation is to recognize the current phase of the surgery using formal knowledge, experience-based knowledge or a combination thereof. A model was built based on the activities which occurred during the surgery and infer the higher level phases, which overarch individual activities. These activities belong together in the medical sense and lead to a specific sub-goal during the surgery. The phases are defined in such way that each phase is in need of a specific assistance. Thus, knowing the phase, it is possible to automatically use the appropriate subset of available information. This way, the automatic information filtering is realized. The information about which activities occurred is assumed as given. The detection of these is outside of the scope of this work.

Methodically, formal knowledge about the relationship between activities and phases was captured with rules. The rules are used to check whether the model of the situation satisfies certain conditions which are indicative of a phase, namely Validness and Phase Specificness. The Validness refers to whether there is a valid transition between one phase to another. A transition is called valid if it does not contradict the surgery plan. The Phase Specificness refers to whether there is an activity in the current model which is strongly connected to and indicative of the beginning of a specific phase. Such activities are called Triggering Activities.

Several rule languages were used for this purpose, namely nRQL, SWRL, ad-hoc rules with OWL API and SQWRL. Although none satisfied all of the requirements, SQWRL came very close. It only lacked in tool support. As the field matures, this issue is likely to be resolved.

For the experience-based approach the Random Forest algorithm was used to realize phase recognition and nGrams for the prediction of activities. Both algorithms rely solely on experience-based knowledge.

To combine the complementary approaches two methods were developed: formal approach was augmented with experience and the experience-based approach with formal knowledge. To augment the formal knowledge based approach with experience, rules were learned from annotated surgeries. The idea is to distill the parts relevant for situation interpretation into an explicit, human-readable form. This captures tacit knowledge, given that it is contained in the experience. The resulting rules can then be verified, extended and corrected by medical experts as necessary. Thus, experience-based knowledge is transferred to formal knowledge. It is made explicit and formalized. Methodically, the approach is inspired by the paradigm of swarm optimization.

To enhance the experience with formal knowledge, a so-called Composition of Random Forests was developed. The (formal) knowledge about possible transitions of phases given by the surgery plan is exploited to partition the task of phase recognition over multiple Random Forests so that each Random Forest only has to consider a limited number of phases.

It is hard to rank the proposed methods by the quality measures which were investigated (recognition rate, confusion matrix, variance and runtime). The division between the algorithms is not along the lines of the type of knowledge they use, but whether they are rule-based or not. The rule-based approaches, either with rules extracted from medical experts or automatically from experience-based knowledge, perform very well on undistorted data. However, they are not robust against noise.

Machine-learning approaches, based on experience-based knowledge are robust. They are only slightly affected by noise. Yet their recognition rates are lower in the undistorted case. More severely, in the evaluation they were not always capable of recognizing all phases. It is likely that this is caused by too few samples. Given additional annotated surgeries, the results of the machine-learning based approaches could improve. This explains why there were more problems with short phases than with longer ones. For short phases, there was less training data available.

Context-Aware Augmented Reality in Laparascopy and Dental Implant Surgery The phase recognition is used to infer the current phase of the surgery. With this information, the appropriate subset of available information is presented to the surgeon. For this purpose, Augmented Reality visualizations were developed. In the laparascopic use-case, the focus is on the visualization of targets (e.g. tumors) and vital structures (e.g. veins). The Augmented Reality images for this use-case are displayed in the endoscopic images. This is the view surgeons are already accustomed to. It can be delivered with monitors already present in regular operating rooms. For dental implants visual assistance about the correct placing and aligning of the dental bur in the mandible is provided. The visualizations are shown using a head mounted display to better fit in the established workflow of the procedure.

To evaluate the application to Laparascopy, a system for context-aware assistance of pancreatic resections was developed. Assistance in finding the target structure, resecting diseased tissue and warnings when vital structure were endangered was provided. The system was evaluated on a silicon liver phantom. Furthermore, a system which warns the surgeon in case of risky situations during removals of the gallbladder was developed. This system was evaluated on a porcine liver. For this to work, a method which inferred activities from distance measurements was developed. This was necessary as it was the only input given by the underlying assistance system. The solution is based on mapping of numerical measurements to qualitative labels using fuzzy sets.

For the evaluation in case of dental implant surgery the drilling of implant position was performed in the mandible of a porcine head. The aim was to realize implant positions, while information was selectively displayed only about the implant position currently being worked on. The visualizations have been shown on a see-through head mounted display. This device needs special calibration. A novel calibration protocol for it has been proposed and implemented.

The evaluation shows that context-awareness has great potential in improving surgical practices. Particularly, it is likely to make surgeries easier and less risky to perform. The surgeon can focus on his patient, receive important hints and pieces of information without being disturbed by assistance devices. Assistance systems automatically adapting to the needs and workflows of the surgeon are very be beneficial. Although the evaluations highly suggest that these claims are true, they could not be proven. The final proof is still open and cannot be found in current literature.

To actually arrive at such a result, more studies are necessary to show statistically significant improvements in quality parameters such as surgeon fatigue, duration of the surgery and patient outcome. Such large-scale studies are beyond the scope of this thesis.

9.2. Outlook

The research of this work can be extended to a wide range of application. Particularly, the knowledge representation is versatile.

The representation of the surgery in this work is restricted to phases and activities. However, there is a large amount of additional data that could be incorporated in the model. For instance, it could be extended to not only consider the actions of the surgeon, but also those of other surgical staff, like nurses and anesthesiologist. Additionally, speech acts, like giving orders and asking for information, could be included to cover verbal interaction between the staff.

Further Development of the Knowledge Representation In addition to information on the human actors, the data from medical devices could be integrated into the representation. Initiatives like the integrated operating room OR1 made by Storz, for instance, plays a major part in this endeavor. Such systems provide easy access to device parameters and outputs which could be modeled in LapOntoSPM and The Ontology for Laparascopy to be part of the description of workflows.

Another aspects of surgical workflows apart from human actors and medical devices are algorithms and data structures. They are part of the surgical workflow, as they influence behavior and decision making. The extension of the ontology to include medical data and algorithms can help to better understand the workflow.

New Application Scenarios Apart from the intraoperative use, the formal and experience-based knowledge can be applied to optimize workflows. The idea in this case is to provide suggestion on which course of action is likely to improve efficiency and outcome. This could be done, for instance by defining gold standards of how surgeries should be done and how certain situation are best handled. If deviations from these best practices are detected, cues could be offered to the surgeon. This can lead to post-operative evaluation of the surgery to asses the expertise of the surgeon. Similarity measures which make use of the formal and experience-based knowledge to compare a given workflow can be used to compare given surgical workflows to the gold standards.

Broader Scope While this work is strictly focused on intraoperative scenarios, similar methods can be applied also to post- and preoperative therapy. The entire treatment of the patient, from stepping into a hospital, over diagnosis, surgical therapy to postoperative treatment can be modeled as a process, similar to the intraoperative one. The model of the surgical process, as described in this work would then be part of an overarching description of the entire therapy and diagnosis of the patient. Then similar interpretation algorithms could be used to identify critical points of the treatment to offer targeted assistance or to optimize the workflow.

A. Formalization of Surgeries

Phases of Pancreatic Resections

Phase	Description
Start	Beginning of the intervention
Port placement	Insertion of surgical instruments and the endoscope
Mobilisation	Transsection of the gastrocolic ligament access the pancreas.
Dissection	Dissection of the parietal peritoneum to mobilize the pancreas
Resection	Removal of pathologic tissue of the pancreas (e.g. IPMN, benign tumor or cyst)
Closure	Removal of resected tissue in a specimen bag
Drain	Drainage for early indication of pancreatic fistula or bleeding

Figure A.1.: Phases of pancreas resection

Triggering Activities of Pancreatic Resections

Phase	Triggering Activities
Start	-
Port placement	(Port, place, Abdomen)
Mobilisation	(AtraumaticGrasper, grasp, GastrocolicLigament), (Instr, surgicalAction, splenocolicLigament), (AtraumaticGrasper, grasp, GreaterOmentum), (SharpInstr, cuttingAction, GastrocolicLigament), (SharpInstr, cuttingAction, Adhesion)
Dissection	(SharpInstr, cuttingAction, DorsalParietalPeritoneum), (Instrument, bluntDissect, DorsalParietalPeritoneum), (AtraumaticGrasper grasp DorsalParietalPeritoneum), (BluntInstr, bluntDissect, SplenicArtery), (SharpInstr, dissect, SplenicArtery), (Clip, clipping, SplenicArtery), (Instr, knot, SplenicArtery), (BluntInstr, bluntDissect, SplenicVein), (SharpInstr, dissect, SplenicVein), (Clip, clipping, SplenicVein), (Instr, knot, SplenicVein)
Resection	(SharpInstr, cuttingAction, Pancreas), (SharpInstr, cuttingAction, RetropancreaticTissue), (SharpInstr, dissect, Pancreas), (SharpInstr, cuttingAction, Tumor), (SharpInstr, cuttingAction, Cyst), (Stapler, resect, Pancreas), (NeedleHolder, suture, Pancreas), (NeedleHolder, suture, Stomach), (SharpInstr, cuttingAction, SplenicArtery), (SharpInstr, cuttingAction, SplenicVein)
Closure	(SpecimenBag, surgicalAction, Organ)
Drain	(Drainage, surgicalAction, organ)

Figure A.2.: Triggering activities of pancreas resection

Valid Phase Transitions for Pancreatic Resection

	resection	mobilisation	start	dissection	closure	drain	port placement
resection	X	X		X	X	X	X
mobilisation	X	X		X		X	X
start		X	X				X
dissection	X	X		X			X
closure	X	X			X	X	
drain						X	
port placement		X		X		X	X

X = valid transition between phases

Figure A.3.: Valid transitions of pancreas resection

Phases of Adrenalectomy

Phase	Description
Start	Begin of the surgery
Port placement	Insertion of surgical instruments and the endoscope
Mobilisation	Mobilization of adjacent adhesions and the colon to access gerota's fascia
Dissection	Cutting of gerota's fascia to get direct access to the adrenal gland
Resection	Resection of the adrenal gland
Closure	Removal of adrenal gland in a specimen bag
Drain	Drainage for an early indication of bleeding

Figure A.4.: Phases of Adrenalectomy

Triggering Activities of Adrenalectomies

Phase	Triggering Activities
Start	-
Port placement	(port, place, abdomen)
Mobilisation	(SharpInstr, cuttingAction, Adhesion), (SharpInstr, mobilize, Liver), (AtraumaticGrasper, lift, Liver), (AtraumaticGrasper, grasp, Adhesion), (AtraumaticGrasper, grasp, GreaterOmentum), (SharpInstr, cuttingAction, SplenoralLigament), (SharpInstr, mobilize, Colon)
Dissection	(SharpInstr, cuttingAction, GerotasFascia), (Instr, surgicalAction, DorsalParietalPeritoneum)
Resection	(SharpInstr, cuttingAction, AdrenalGland), (Instr, surgicalAction, PerirenalFatTissue)
Closure	(SpecimenBag, surgicalAction, organ), (AtraumaticGrasper, puttingAction, ResectedTissue)
Drain	(Drainage, surgicalAction, organ)

Figure A.5.: Triggering activities of adrenalectomy

Valid Phase Transitions for Adrenalectomy

	resection	mobilisation	start	dissection	closure	drain	port placement
resection	×			×	×		
mobilisation		×		×			×
start		×	×				×
dissection	×	×		×			×
closure					×	×	
drain						×	
port placement	×	×		×			×

× valid transition between phases

Figure A.6.: Valid transitions of adrenalectomy

Phases for Cholecystectomies

Phase	Description
Start	Begin of the surgery
Port placement	Insertion of surgical instruments and the endoscope
Mobilisation	Exposure of the gallbladder
Dissection	Prepationduring of the triangle of calot
Resection cystic artery	Resection of the the cystic artery
Resection cystic duct	Resection of the cystic duct
Resection gallbladder	Removal of the gallbladder from the liverbed
Closure	Removal of the gallbladder in a specimen bag
Drain	Drainage of infectious liquid or for early indication of bleeding

Figure A.7.: Phases of Cholecystectomy

Triggering Activities for Cholecystectomies

Phase	Triggering Activities
Start	-
Port placement	(Port, place, Abdomen)
Mobilisation	(AtraumaticGrasper, grasp, GallbladderFundus), (AtraumaticGrasper, grasp, GastrocolicLigament)
Dissection	(AtraumaticGrasper, grasp ,HepatoduodenalLigament), (AtraumaticGrasper, lift , HepatoduodenalLigament), (Instr, surgicalAction, CalotTriangle), (SharpInstr, cuttingAction, HepatoduodenalLigament)
Resection cystic artery	(SharpInstr, cut, CysticArtery), (Clip, clipping, CysticArtery)
Resection cystic duct	(SharpInstr, cuttingAction, CysticDuct), (Clip, clipping, CysticDuct)
Resection gallbladder	(SharpInstr, cuttingAction, GallbladderSerosa), (SharpInstr, dissect, GallbladderSerosa), (SharpInstr, cuttingAction, Gallbladder), (SharpInstr, cuttingAction, GallbladderLiverbed)
Closure	(SpecimenBag, surgicalAction, Organ)
Drain	(Drainage, surgicalAction, organ)

Figure A.8.: Triggering activities of Cholecystectomy

Valid Phase Transitions for Cholecystectomies

	resection_cystic_artery	mobilisation	start	dissection	closure	drain	resection_cystic_duct	port_placement	resection_gallbladder
resection_cystic_artery	×						×		×
mobilisation		×		×					
start		×	×	×				×	×
dissection	×			×			×		×
closure					×	×			
drain						×			
resection_cystic_duct	×						×		×
port_placement		×		×				×	
resection_gallbladder				×	×				×

☒ valid transition between phases

Figure A.9.: Valid transitions of Cholecystectomy

Bibliography

[1] E.C. Adam. Fighter cockpits of the future. In , *AIAA/IEEE Digital Avionics Systems Conference, 1993. 12th DASC*, pages 318–323, 1993.

[2] S.A. Ahmadi, T. Sielhorst, R. Stauder, M. Horn, H. Feussner, and N. Navab. Recovery of Surgical Workflow Without Explicit Models. In *Medical Image Computing and Computer-Assisted Intervention - MICCAI 2006*, number 4190 in Lecture Notes in Computer Science, pages 420–428. Springer Berlin Heidelberg, 2006.

[3] A. Asuncion and D.J. Newman. UCI Machine Learning Repository.

[4] Franz Baader, Diego Calvanese, Deborah L. McGuinness, Daniele Nardi, and Peter F. Patel-Schneider, editors. *The Description Logic Handbook: Theory, Implementation, and Applications.* Cambridge University Press, New York, NY, USA, 2003.

[5] T. Blum, H. Feußner, and N. Navab. Modeling and Segmentation of Surgical Workflow from Laparoscopic Video. In *Medical Image Computing and Computer-Assisted Intervention - MICCAI 2010*, number 6363 in Lecture Notes in Computer Science, pages 400–407. Springer Berlin Heidelberg, 2010.

[6] L. Bouarfa, P. P. Jonker, and J. Dankelman. Discovery of high-level tasks in the operating room. *Journal of Biomedical Informatics*, 44(3):455–462, 2011.

[7] L. Breiman. Random Forests. *Machine Learning*, 45(1):5–32, 2001.

[8] K. Cleary, A. Kinsella, and S.K. Mun. OR 2020 workshop report: Operating room of the future. *International Congress Series*, 1281:832–838, 2005.

[9] O. Corcho, M. Fernández-López, and A. Gómez-Pérez. Methodologies, Tools and Languages for Building Ontologies: Where is Their Meeting Point? *Data Knowl. Eng.*, 46(1):41–64, 2003.

[10] B.J. Dixon, M.J. Daly, H. Chan, A.D. Vescan, I.J. Witterick, and J.C. Irish. Surgeons blinded by enhanced navigation: the effect of augmented reality on attention. *Surgical Endoscopy*, 27(2):454–461, 2013.

[11] G. Forestier, L. Riffaud, and P. Jannin. Automatic phase prediction from low-level surgical activities. *International Journal of Computer Assisted Radiology and Surgery*, 10(6):833–841, 2015.

[12] S. Franke, J. Meixensberger, and T. Neumuth. Multi-perspective workflow modeling for online surgical situation models. *Journal of Biomedical Informatics*, 54:158–166, 2015.

[13] B. Gibaud, C. Penet, and P. Jannin. OntoSPM: a core ontology of surgical procedure models. In *Surgetica*, 2014.

[14] V. Haarslev, K. Hidde, R. Möller, and M. Wessel. The Racerpro Knowledge Representation and Reasoning System. *Semant. web*, 3(3):267–277, 2012.

[15] M. Horridge and S. Bechhofer. The OWL API: A Java API for OWL Ontologies. *Semant. web*, 2(1):11–21, 2011.

[16] P. Jannin and X. Morandi. Surgical models for computer-assisted neurosurgery. *NeuroImage*, 37(3):783–791, 2007.

[17] J.P. Joyce and G.W. Lapinsky. A History and Overview of the Safety Parameter Display System Concept. *IEEE Transactions on Nuclear Science*, 30(1):744–749, 1983.

[18] D. Katić, S. Brandstädter, A.L. Wekerle, H. Kenngott, B.P. Müller-Stich, R. Dillmann, and S. Speidel. Knowledge-Based Approach for a Context-Aware Augmented Reality Assistance System. In *Proceedings of KogWis*, 2012.

[19] D. Katić, G. Castrillon-Oberndorfer, G. Sudra, S. Speidel, G. Eggers, and R. Dillmann. Wissensbasierter Ansatz zur kontextbezogenen Erweiterten Realität in der Dentalimplantologie. In *Computer- und Roboterassistierte Chirurgie (CURAC)*, 2010.

[20] D. Katić, T. Christian, G. Castrillon-Oberndorfer, J. Hoffmann, G. Eggers, R. Dillmann, and S. Speidel. Calibration of see-through Goggles for a context-aware augmented reality system. In *Computer Assisted Radiology and Surgery (CARS)*, 2011.

[21] D. Katić, C. Julliard, A.L. Wekerle, H. Kenngott, B.P. Müller-Stich, R. Dillmann, S. Speidel, P. Jannin, and B. Gibaud. LapOntoSPM: an ontology for laparoscopic surgeries and its application to surgical phase recognition. *International Journal of Computer Assisted Radiology and Surgery*, 2015.

[22] D. Katić, J. Schuck, A.L. Wekerle, H. Kenngott, B.P. Mueller-Stich, D. Ruediger, and S. Speidel. Robust situation interpretation with a composition of random forests and ontological background knowledge. In *MICCAI Workshop M2CAI*, 2015.

[23] D. Katić, P. Spengler, S. Bodenstedt, G. Castrillon-Oberndorfer, R. Seeberger, J. Hoffmann, R. Dillmann, and S. Speidel. Ein System zur situationsbezogenen Unterstützung in der Dentalimplantologie. In *Bildverarbeitung für die Medizin 2014*, Informatik aktuell, pages 348–353. Springer Berlin Heidelberg, 2014.

[24] D. Katić, G. Sudra, S. Speidel, G. Castrillon-Oberndorfer, G. Eggers, and R. Dillmann. Context-aware Augmented Reality for Dental Implant Surgery, Proc. Computer Assisted Radiology and Surgery. In *Computer Assisted Radiology and Surgery (CARS)*, 2010.

[25] D. Katić, G. Sudra, S. Speidel, G. Castrillon-Oberndorfer, G. Eggers, and R. Dillmann. Knowledge-Based Situation Interpretation for Context-Aware Augmented Reality in Dental Implant Surgery. In *Medical Imaging and Augmented Reality*, number 6326 in Lecture Notes in Computer Science, pages 531–540. Springer Berlin Heidelberg, 2010.

[26] D. Katić, A.L. Wekerle, S. Bodenstedt, H. Kenngott, B.P. Müller-Stich, R. Dillmann, and S. Speidel. Logic-Based Situation Interpretation with Real-Valued Sensor Data for Laparoscopic Surgery. In *MICCAI Workshop on Modeling and Monitoring of Computer Assisted Interventions (M2CAI)*, 2011.

[27] D. Katić, A.L. Wekerle, F. Gärtner, H. Kenngott, B.P. Müller-Stich, R. Dillmann, and S. Speidel. Ontology-based prediction of surgical events in laparoscopic surgery. In *SPIE Medical Imaging*, volume 8671, page 86711A, 2013.

[28] D. Katić, A.L. Wekerle, F. Gärtner, H. Kenngott, B.P. Müller-Stich, R. Dillmann, and S. Speidel. Knowledge-driven formalization of laparoscopic surgeries for rule-based intraoperative context-aware assistance. In *Information Processing in Computer-Assisted Interventions*, pages 158–167. Springer International Publishing, 2014.

[29] D. Katić, A.L. Wekerle, F. Gärtner, H. Kenngott, B.P. Müller-Stich, R. Dillmann, and S. Speidel. Model-based formalization of medical knowledge for context-aware assistance in laparoscopic surgery. In *SPIE Medical Imaging*, volume 9036, page 903603, 2014.

[30] D. Katić, A.L. Wekerle, J. Görtler, P. Spengler, S. Bodenstedt, S. Röhl, S. Suwelack, H.G. Kenngott, M. Wagner, B.P. Müller-Stich, R. Dillmann, and S. Speidel. Context-aware Augmented Reality in laparoscopic surgery. *Computerized Medical Imaging and Graphics*, 37(2):174–182, 2013.

[31] J. Kennedy and R. Eberhart. Particle swarm optimization. In *, IEEE International Conference on Neural Networks, 1995. Proceedings*, volume 4, pages 1942–1948 vol.4, 1995.

[32] Z. Kobti, R. G. Reynolds, and T. Kohler. Agent-Based Modeling of Cultural Change in Swarm Using Cultural Algorithms. In *Swarmfest04*, 2004.

[33] M. Kranzfelder, C. Staub, A. Fiolka, A. Schneider, S. Gillen, D. Wilhelm, H. Friess, A. Knoll, and H. Feussner. Toward increased autonomy in the surgical OR: needs, requests, and expectations. *Surgical Endoscopy*, 27(5):1681–1688, 2013.

[34] S. Kripalani, R. Bengtzen, L.E. Henderson, and T.A. Jacobson. Clinical research in low-literacy populations: using teach-back to assess comprehension of informed consent and privacy information. *IRB*, 30(2):13–19, 2008.

[35] F. Lalys, D. Bouget, L. Riffaud, and P. Jannin. Automatic knowledge-based recognition of low-level tasks in ophthalmological procedures. *International Journal of Computer Assisted Radiology and Surgery*, 8(1):39–49, 2013.

[36] F. Lalys and P. Jannin. Surgical process modelling: a review. *International Journal of Computer Assisted Radiology and Surgery*, 9(3):495–511, 2014.

[37] F. Lalys, L. Riffaud, D. Bouget, and P. Jannin. A framework for the recognition of high-level surgical tasks from video images for cataract surgeries. *IEEE transactions on bio-medical engineering*, 59(4):966–976, 2012.

[38] F. Lalys, L. Riffaud, X. Morandi, and P. Jannin. Surgical Phases Detection from Microscope Videos by Combining SVM and HMM. In *Medical Computer Vision. Recognition Techniques and Applications in Medical Imaging*, number 6533 in Lecture Notes in Computer Science, pages 54–62. Springer Berlin Heidelberg, 2011.

[39] C.A. Linte, K.P. Davenport, K. Cleary, C. Peters, K.G. Vosburgh, N. Navab, P.E. Edwards, P. Jannin, T.M. Peters, D.R. Holmes, and R.A. Robb. On mixed reality environments for minimally invasive therapy guidance: systems architecture, successes and challenges in their implementation from laboratory to clinic. *Computerized Medical Imaging and Graphics: The Official Journal of the Computerized Medical Imaging Society*, 37(2):83–97, 2013.

[40] H. Ma and Y. Wang. Cultural Algorithm Based on Particle Swarm Optimization for Function Optimization. In *Fifth International Conference on Natural Computation, 2009. ICNC '09*, volume 3, pages 224–228, 2009.

[41] M. Mohri, A. Rostamizadeh, and A. Talwalkar. *Foundations of Machine Learning*. The MIT Press, 2012.

[42] T. Neumuth, P. Jannin, J. Schlomberg, J. Meixensberger, P. Wiedemann, and O. Burgert. Analysis of surgical intervention populations using generic surgical process models. *International Journal of Computer Assisted Radiology and Surgery*, 6(1):59–71, 2011.

[43] T. Neumuth, P. Jannin, G. Strauss, J. Meixensberger, and O. Burgert. Validation of Knowledge Acquisition for Surgical Process Models. *Journal of the American Medical Informatics Association : JAMIA*, 16(1):72–80, 2009.

[44] T. Neumuth, G. Strauß, J. Meixensberger, H.U. Lemke, and O. Burgert. Acquisition of Process Descriptions from Surgical Interventions. In *Database and Expert Systems Applications*, number 4080 in Lecture Notes in Computer Science, pages 602–611. Springer Berlin Heidelberg, 2006.

[45] M. O'Connor and A. Das. SQWRL: a Query Language for OWL. In *OWL: Experiences and Directions*, volume 529, 2009.

[46] M. O'Connor, H. Knublauch, S. Tu, B. Grosof, M. Dean, W. Grosso, and M. Musen. Supporting Rule System Interoperability on the Semantic Web with SWRL. In *The Semantic Web - ISWC 2005*, number 3729 in Lecture Notes in Computer Science, pages 974–986. Springer Berlin Heidelberg, 2005.

[47] C. Rosse and Jose L.V.M. Jr. The Foundational Model of Anatomy Ontology. In *Anatomy Ontologies for Bioinformatics*, number 6 in Computational Biology, pages 59–117. Springer London, 2008.

[48] R. Shearer, B. Motik, and I. Horrocks. HermiT: A Highly-Efficient OWL Reasoner. In *Proc. of the 5th Int. Workshop on OWL: Experiences and Directions (OWLED 2008 EU)*, 2008.

[49] E. Sirin, B. Parsia, B.C. Grau, A. Kalyanpur, and Y. Katz. Pellet: A Practical OWL-DL Reasoner. *Web Semant.*, 5(2):51–53, 2007.

[50] P. Skagestad. Thinking with machines: Intelligence augmentation, evolutionary epistemology, and semiotic. *Journal of Social and Evolutionary Systems*, 16(2):157–180, 1993.

[51] E.E. Smith, C. Langston, and R.E. Nisbett. The case for rules in reasoning. *Cognitive Science*, 16(1):1–40, 1992.

[52] S. Speidel, J. Benzko, S. Krappe, G. Sudra, P. Azad, B.P. Müller-Stich, C. Gutt, and R. Dillmann. Automatic classification of minimally invasive instruments based on endoscopic image sequences. In *SPIE Medical Imaging*, pages 72610A–72610A–8, 2009.

[53] R. Stauder, A. Okur, L. Peter, A. Schneider, M. Kranzfelder, H. Feussner, and N. Navab. Random Forests for Phase Detection in Surgical Workflow Analysis. In *Information Processing in Computer-Assisted Interventions*, number 8498 in Lecture Notes in Computer Science, pages 148–157. Springer International Publishing, 2014.

[54] R. Sun. Commonsense Reasoning with Rules, Cases, and Connectionist Models: A Paradigmatic Comparison. *Fuzzy Sets Syst.*, 82(2):187–200, 1996.

[55] Ron Sun and Frederic Alexandre, editors. *Connectionist-Symbolic Integration: From Unified to Hybrid Approaches.* L. Erlbaum Associates Inc., Hillsdale, NJ, USA, 1997.

[56] Ron Sun and Lawrence A. Bookman, editors. *Computational Architectures Integrating Neural And Symbolic Processes*, volume 292 of *The Springer International Series In Engineering and Computer Science.* Springer US, Boston, MA, 1994.

[57] T. Suzuki, Y. Sakurai, K. Yoshimitsu, K. Nambu, Y. Muragaki, and H. Iseki. Intraoperative multichannel audio-visual information recording and automatic surgical phase and incident detection. *IEEE Engineering in Medicine and Biology Society.*, 2010:1190–1193, 2010.

[58] D. Tsarkov and I. Horrocks. FaCT++ Description Logic Reasoner: System Description. In *Proceedings of the Third International Joint Conference on Automated Reasoning*, IJCAR'06, pages 292–297, Berlin, Heidelberg, 2006. Springer-Verlag.

[59] M. Tuceryan and N. Navab. Single point active alignment method (SPAAM) for optical see-through HMD calibration for AR. In *IEEE and ACM International Symposium on Augmented Reality, 2000. (ISAR 2000). Proceedings*, pages 149–158, 2000.

[60] J. Weisbrod. A New Approach to Fuzzy Reasoning. *Soft Computing*, 2:89–99, 1998.

[61] I. Wolf, M. Vetter, I. Wegner, M. Nolden, T. Böttger, M. Hastenteufel, M. Schöbinger, T. Kunert, and H.P. Meinzer. The Medical Imaging Interaction Toolkit (MITK) - a toolkit facilitating the creation of interactive software by extending VTK and ITK. In *SPIE Medical Imaging*, 2004.

[62] D. D. Woods, E.S. Patterson, E.M. Roth, and K. Christoffersen. Can We Ever Escape From Data Overload? A Cognitive Systems Diagnosis. *Cognition, Technology and Work*, 4:22–36, 2002.

[63] Z. Xiang, M. Courtot, R.R. Brinkman, A. Ruttenberg, and Y. He. OntoFox: web-based support for ontology reuse. *BMC Research Notes*, 3(1):175, 2010.